D1773792

DIET IN PREGNANCY: A RANDOMIZED CONTROLLED TRIAL OF NUTRITIONAL SUPPLEMENTS

BOOKS PUBLISHED BY ALAN R. LISS, INC.
FOR MARCH OF DIMES BIRTH DEFECTS FOUNDATION

Birth Defects Compendium, Second Edition, Daniel Bergsma, *Editor*

BIRTH DEFECTS: ORIGINAL ARTICLE SERIES
1980 — Volume XVI

No. 1   **Enzyme Therapy in Genetic Diseases: 2,** Robert J. Desnick, *Editor*

No. 2   **In Vitro Epithelia and Birth Defects,** B. Shannon Danes, *Editor*

No. 3   **Diet in Pregnancy: A Randomized Controlled Trial of Nutritional Supplements,** by David Rush, Zena Stein, and Mervyn Susser

No. 4   **Morphogenesis and Malformation of the Ear,** Robert J. Gorlin, *Editor*

No. 5   **Dentistry in the Treatment of Genetic Diseases,** Carlos F. Salinas and Ronald J. Jorgenson, *Editors*

See pages 199–200 for other volumes in this series published by Alan R. Liss, Inc.

March of Dimes Birth Defects Foundation
Birth Defects: Original Article Series, Volume XVI, Number 3, 1980

DIET IN PREGNANCY: A RANDOMIZED CONTROLLED TRIAL OF NUTRITIONAL SUPPLEMENTS

David Rush, MD
Columbia University

Zena Stein, MA, MB, BCh
New York Psychiatric Institute
and
Columbia University

Mervyn Susser, MB, BCh, DPH, FRCP(E)
Columbia University

Assitant Editor
Sue Conde Greene
March of Dimes Birth Defects Foundation

ALAN R. LISS, INC., NEW YORK

To enhance medical communication in the birth defects field, the March of Dimes Birth Defects Foundation publishes the *Birth Defects Compendium (Second Edition)*, an *Original Article Series, Syndrome Identification,* a *Reprint Series,* and provides a series of films and related brochures.

Further information can be obtained from:

March of Dimes Birth Defects Foundation
Medical Education Division
1275 Mamaroneck Avenue
White Plains, New York 10605

Published by:

Alan R. Liss, Inc.
150 Fifth Avenue
New York, New York 10011

Copyright ©1980 by March of Dimes Birth Defects Foundation

All rights reserved. No part of this publication may be reproduced or transmitted in any form or by any means, electronic or mechanical, including photocopying and recording, or by any information storage and retrieval system, without permission in writing from the copyright holder.

Views expressed in articles published are the authors', and are not to be attributed to the March of Dimes Birth Defects Foundation or its editors unless expressly so stated.

Library of Congress Cataloging in Publication Data

Rush, David.
    Diet in pregnancy: A randomized controlled
    trial of nutritional supplements.
    (Birth defects original article series; v. 16, no. 3)
    Bibliography: pp. 181–187
    Includes index.
    1. Pregnancy – Nutritional aspects. 2. High-protein
diet. 3. Infants – Growth. 4. Infant psychology. I. Stein,
Zena, joint author. II. Susser, Mervyn W., joint author. III.
Title. IV. Series. [DNLM: 1. Nutrition – In pregnancy. 2.
Prenatal care. W1 BI966 v. 16 no. 3 / WQ175 R952]
RG626.B63 vol. 16, no. 3 [RG559] 616'.043s [618;3'2'05]
ISBN 0-8451-1037-3   79-3846

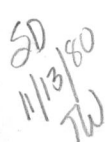

The **MARCH OF DIMES BIRTH DEFECTS FOUNDATION** is dedicated to the goal of preventing birth defects and ameliorating their consequences for patients, families, and society.

As part of our efforts to achieve these goals, we sponsor, or participate in, a variety of scientific meetings and symposia where all questions relating to birth defects are freely discussed. Through our professional educational program we speed the dissemination of information by publishing the proceedings of these meetings and symposia. From time to time, we also reprint pertinent journal articles to help achieve our goal. Now and then, in the course of these articles or discussions, individual viewpoints may be expressed which go beyond the purely scientific and into controversial matters. It should be noted, therefore, that personal viewpoints about such matters will not be censored but this does not constitute an endorsement of them by the **March of Dimes Birth Defects Foundation**.

Contents

Figures xii
Tables xiii
Preface xv
Acknowledgments xxiv
Participating Investigators xxv
Project Staff xxvi

Chapter I. Rationale and Design of the Study, and Enrollment of the Sample
David Rush, Zena Stein, Mervyn Susser, *with* Joseph Fleiss
    Rationale 1
    Design 4
        Sample Size 5
        Target Population and Selection Criteria 5
        Forms of Treatment 9
        Procedures 13
        Outcome Measures 18
    Recruitment, Selection, Attrition 19
    Other Attributes of Treatment Groups 20
    Conclusion 24
    Summary 24

Chapter II. The Monitoring of Experimental Intervention
    Monitoring 27
        Indices of Adherence to Treatment: Description ... 28
            Quantitative 24-hour dietary recall 28
            Direct structured questioning 28
            Inventory of unused beverage (can count) 28
            Urinary riboflavin assay 29

viii / Contents

Indices of Adherence to Treatment: Interrelationships	29
Diet Intake	30
Intercorrelations of Beverage Intake Indices	30
Estimates of Beverage Intake, and Substitution of Regular Diet	34
Weight Gain	41
Indices of Weight Gain	41
Treatment Effects on Weight Gain	44
Dietary Intake and Weight Gain	45
Discussion and Conclusions	47
Nutritional Intake	47
Weight Gain	49
Summary	53
Chapter III. Outcome at Birth: Effects on Duration of Gestation, Mortality, and Size	
Results	55
Duration of Gestation	55
Dietary intake and extreme prematurity	57
Duration of gestation and maternal characteristics	57
Perinatal Mortality	58
Characteristics of pregnancies ending in perinatal death	60
Fetal Growth and Size at Birth	61
Birthweight and treatment	64
Birthweight, treatment, and entry cohort	65
Birthweight, treatment, and maturity	65
Birthweight, maturity, and entry cohort	66
Treatment effects on newborn dimensions	67
Dietary indices and newborn dimensions	67
Control variables and conditional effects	69
Newborn dimensions and smoking	72
Newborn dimensions and past low birthweight	74
Discussion	75
Between-Group Differences: Outcome	75
Within-Group Differences: Process	78
Adverse effects of the high protein Supplement	80
Conclusion	83
Summary	85

Chapter IV. Outcome at One Year of Age: Effects on Somatic and Psychological Measures
David Rush, Zena Stein, Mervyn Susser, *with* Nathan Brody
   Methods and Procedures 88
      Testing Procedures 89
      Rationale for Choice of Measures............. 91
   Results.................................... 92
      Somatic Measures and Treatment............. 92
      Psychological Measures and Treatment 93
      Control of Confounding 96
      Some Regression Analyses.................. 96
      Treatment, Premature Birth, and Outcome 97
   Discussion 97
      The Meaning of the Protein-Related Measures.... 99
      Protein Levels and Protein-Related Measures 101
      One-Year Outcome and Adverse Outcome at Birth 102
      Conclusion 103
      Summary 103

Chapter V. Prenatal Nutritional, Quasi, and Natural Experiments in the Past Decade: An Overview
   Introduction 105
      The New York Study 107
      The Montreal Study 108
      The Bogotá Study 110
      The Guatemala Study 112
      The Taiwan Study....................... 117
      The Dutch Famine Study.................. 120
   Conclusions 123
      Birthweight 123
      Psychological Effects 125
         With regard to the usual "growth-related" measures of psychological development 131
         With regard to the "protein-related" measures of psychological development 131

Appendices

    1.1. Information Collected on Participants During Pregnancy 133

1.2. Information Collected on Participants at Delivery and Follow-Up 134
2.1. Three Indices of Weight Gain by Treatment and Entry Cohort:
   a. All deliveries 135
   b. Deliveries < 37 weeks gestation 136
   c. Deliveries 37+ weeks gestation 137
2.2a. Early Weight Gain and Treatment: Multiple regression analysis 138
   b. Early Weight Gain and Treatment: Multiple regression analysis 139
   c. Average Weight Gain and Treatment: Multiple regression analysis 140
   d. Average Weight Gain and Treatment: Multiple regression analysis 141
   e. Average Weight Gain and Diet Intake: Multiple regression analysis 142
3.1. Treatment and Prematurity: Life table analysis 143
3.2. Treatment and Neonatal Death: Life table analysis 144
3.3. Individual Data on Neonatal Death: Selected characteristics of mothers, pregnancies, and their infants, for each neonatal death by treatment group among participants active to delivery 145
3.4. Newborn Dimensions, Weight Gain, Diet, and Smoking 147
3.5a. Birthweight and Treatment: Multiple regression analysis 149
   b. Birthweight and Treatment: Multiple regression analysis 150
   c. Birthweight and Treatment: Multiple regression analysis 151
   d. Birthweight and Treatment: Multiple regression analysis 152
   e. Birthweight and Diet Intake: Multiple regression analysis 153
4.1. Psychological Indices at Age One 154
4.2. Correlations of Somatic and Psychological Indices 155

4.3.	Somatic Indices at Age One	158
4.4.	Psychological Indices at Age One	161
4.5a.	Bayley Mental Score and Treatment: Multiple regression analysis.	167
b.	Bayley Motor Score and Treatment: Multiple regression analysis	168
c.	Habituation and Treatment: Multiple regression analysis	169
d.	Dishabituation and Treatment: Multiple regression analysis	170
e.	Duration of Episodes of Play and Treatment: Multiple regression analysis	171
5.1.	Summary of Studies of Maternal Nutrition Intervention in Pregnancy	172
6.	Placental Biochemistry and Treatment David Rush, Zena Stein, Mervyn Susser, *with* Myron Winick, Pedro Rosso, Mary Campbell Brown	178
7.	Placental Histomorphometry and Treatment David Rush, Zena Stein, Mervyn Susser, *with* Richard Naeye	178
8.	Histopathology of Placenta David Rush, Zena Stein, Mervyn Susser, *with* William Blanc, Prem Chauhan, Carlos Navarro	180

References ... 181
Index ... 189

FIGURES

Chapter I
1.1. Sequence of procedures for women registering for prenatal care..................... 14
1.2. Retention and Attrition. Survival in the study through pregnancy and the newborn period among all women recruited 21

Chapter II
2.1. Estimates of intake supplied by beverages, among entry cohorts, according to several indices 39
2.2. Estimates of total daily diet intake among entry cohorts for each treatment group....... 40

Chapter III
3.1. Treatment and Prematurity. Cumulative rates of delivery (%) from life tables for each treatment group 56
3.2. Treatment and Neonatal Death. Cumulative rates of neonatal death (%) from life tables for each treatment group.................. 64
3.3. Birthweight in Supplement (S), Complement (C), and Control (contr) groups among premature and mature deliveries 65
3.4 Birthweight in Supplement (S), Complement (C), and Control (contr) groups among women who were smokers, and among women with previous deliveries of low birthweight infants . . 75

TABLES

Chapter I	1.1.	Composition of Daily Diet Supplements for Each Treatment Group.	10
	1.2.	Retention and Attrition	22
	1.3.	Characteristics of Study Population	22
Chapter II	2.1.	Indices of Beverage Intake	31
	2.2.	Validation of Anamnestic Indices of Compliance With Treatment	33
	2.3.	Diet Intake During Study by Treatment Group.	35
	2.4.	Caloric Intake	37
	2.5.	Protein Intake	38
	2.6.	Beverage Intake by Stage of Gestation at Entry to Study	42
	2.7.	Beverage Use by Prior Maternal Characteristics	43
	2.8.	Weight Gain and Dietary Intake	46
Chapter III	3.1.	Dietary and Beverage Intake and Prematurity	59
	3.2.	Prematurity and Relative Protein Levels	60
	3.3.	Duration of Gestation and Antecedent Maternal Factors	61
	3.4.	Treatment and Perinatal Deaths	62
	3.5.	Fetal and Neonatal Mortality Compared	63
	3.6.	Mean Birthweight by Treatment Group in Variously Defined Experimental Groups	68
	3.7.	Birthweight, Treatment, and Entry Cohort	70
	3.8.	Birthweight, Treatment, and Maturity	71
	3.9.	Birthweight, Treatment, Maturity, and Stage of Gestation at Entry	73
	3.10.	Treatment Effects on Selected Newborn Dimensions	74
	3.11.	Summary of Results by Treatment Group	76
Chapter IV	4.1.	Somatic Measures at One Year of Age by Treatment	93
	4.2.	Psychological Measures at One Year of Age by Treatment	94
Chapter V	5.1.	Ten Recent or Ongoing Studies	106
	5.2.	Montreal Study.	109
	5.3.	Bogotá Study	111
	5.4.	Guatemala Study	114
	5.5.	Taiwan Study: Mean Birthweight in Grams (± SD)	119

Preface

This volume comprises the main body of results relating to the central hypothesis of a large intervention study. The diet of pregnant women was supplemented with the aim of improving the growth and development of their offspring both prenatally and through the first year of life.

The volume is a slim one. Its slenderness is not the result of compression or lack of data. In poetry much substance can be distilled from the allusions and connotations of few words. Communicating in that mode is not in the gift of science. The precision we seek and the substance we convey are immeasurably different, and numbers and tables abound in the book. We might find other justifications. In busy times, a book which says what it must in short compass can please. Yet if brevity alone is the aim, we must admit that the material reported here can be cut and shrivelled into a single article.

Our main object in going into book form, despite our few pages, is a different one. Many of the conclusions we reach, on a topic of undeniable public health and medical import, are controversial. In such a case readers, for our sake and theirs, need to be given data sufficient to convince them of the validity of our results and inferences. That amount of information cannot be condensed into a single article. To publish several articles in a journal, on the other hand, is not readily achieved. Respected and widely read journals are inundated with worthy articles seeking publication. Editors are reluctant even to consider printing in a single volume the minimum material needed for an adequate report of a study such as this. Some will offer a supplement at a cost far beyond the resources of most authors. In this instance, Dr. R.J. Haggerty, after having the articles reviewed for *Pediatrics* and finding them acceptable and even important, suggested we resolve the problem of space by abstracting the main findings of each article for the journal and publishing the full series of articles as a monograph. This is the path we followed.*

Why do we consider the study important and why do we anticipate controversy?

The study seems important to us because it addresses hypotheses and a set of assumptions about prenatal nutrition that have both theoretical significance and profound implications for the health, well-being, and competence of children born into poverty, in the developing as well as in the developed world. Serious nutritional deprivation, we know, retards fetal growth and adds to early infant mortality. This result accords with experimental work in animals. More refined hypotheses also flow from the experiments. At the critical or vulnerable period of the brain growth spurt, nutritional deprivation invariably depleted brain cells, slowed brain growth and, it seemed, might retard subsequent development, especially mental development. Here was a nutritional hypothesis, many held, that could help to explain the widespread association of depressed cognitive competence with poverty. Hundreds of millions of people in the less developed world might be affected, and millions in the developed world.

Our parallel study of young men whose mothers were exposed in the third trimester to the Dutch hunger winter of 1944/45, however, found no residual effects on cognition, physique, or health that could be explained by a critical period hypothesis of prenatal nutrition, excepting an effect on the frequency of obesity. A number of alternative explanations of this absence of detectable impact of late prenatal exposure could not be entirely eliminated. One of these explanations, relevant to the study reported in this book, was that effects early in life were compensated for and abolished by later postnatal

---

*Pediatrics (Vol. 65, April 1980) presents a summary version of this monograph together with commentaries by Drs. Howard N. Jacobson, Lewis A. Barness, and Mark Hegsted.

experience. The current study (conceived about the same time) set out to examine the effects of improved prenatal nutrition on the child, from birth through the first year of life.

To study supplementation was by implication to examine the effects of nutritional deprivation, since the target population was widely assumed to suffer from nutritional deficiencies. Preliminary work in the community supported that assumption. In our attempts at mounting definitive studies of the effects of prenatal nutrition, this study adopted the experimental approach. By this means we aimed at once both to establish the causal pathway and to test the possibilities of prevention. Even if we had felt secure about the effects of nutritional deprivation in our population, one could not have taken for granted the success of nutritional intervention. Many variables will usually interact to cause a given outcome. Interventions select one or a few of these, and the effect on the given outcome is of necessity uncertain.

The nutrient most generally implicated in growth and brain development by animal experimental studies of nutrient deficiencies was protein. Protein was therefore the main focus of the intervention. To achieve a double-blind design we compared a high protein supplement to one with balanced protein and calorie content. The results of such an experimental study in a human population clearly have bearing both on biological theory about physical and mental growth and development, and on the promotion of health for multitudes.

So much for the importance of this study. We anticipate the results will be controversial because they do not support many of our initial assumptions, assumptions we shared with many scientists well-established in the fields of nutrition and human development. First, it turned out that the deprived black population we studied in New York was not protein deprived as preliminary work had led us to expect and as prevailing opinion held. By United States' standards, the deficiency in the diet of the women recruited was one of calories. Whether their nutritional state pointed to error in our initial assumptions, or to a change in diet owed to widespread social and food programs introduced in the 1960's, we cannot say. Sound data on the question prior to the beginning of this study are not available.

Fortunately, the study was not vitiated and the population remained an appropriate target. Pregnant women in this community continued as before at high risk of bearing low birthweight infants. A decline in the risk of low birthweight did occur in the late 1960's and thereafter. Some of the decline can be attributed to the liberalization of legislation on abortion, and some probably to improvement in social and nutritional conditions. But the high risk of low birthweight in the population was far from being removed.

Second, the effect of protein supplements in this study runs contrary to prevailing assumptions. The conclusion that high protein supplementation had an adverse effect on some women's pregnancies is difficult to deny. Existing nutritional theory does not enable us to advance a reasonable explanation for this outcome. The conclusion is painful, not the least to ourselves. One can be sure that it will be attacked, explained away as a chance finding, or attributed to error, to a toxic contaminant, to racism, and to many less likely causes.

Third, as expected, the high protein supplement, when begun in the first trimester, accelerated maternal weight gain during pregnancy, and maternal weight gain is strongly related to birthweight (as we ourselves showed in preliminary studies). Yet the supplement did not have a favorable effect on birthweight. On the other hand, the balanced protein-calorie supplement diet did not significantly influence maternal weight gain. We have provided a great deal of evidence that the supplements were consumed at an excellent rate. Those who find our interpretation of the results unpalatable, however, may choose to use the selective and conditional relationship of supplementation to accelerated weight gain as evidence of deficient consumption.

Fourth, at the outset of our study we overestimated the potential effect of supplementation. Our review of a number of related studies shows that supplementation produced modest increases in birthweight, of the order of 40 to 70 gm, that is, 2% or less. If there was any effect of either form of supplementation on birthweight, it was too small to reach statistical significance.* The prevalent view, to which we have doubtless contributed, is that there should be a more notable effect.

Fifth, the high protein supplement, but not the balanced protein/calorie supplement, did have effects on special aspects of mental development at one year of age. These effects were remarkable in that they bore no relationship to measures of fetal and infant growth, nor to those measures of psychological development associated with advancing age and physical development. This did not conform to the strongest hypothesis. It is true that in framing hypotheses at the outset of this study, we had allowed for such a contingency. We included a causal pathway passing directly from nutritional supplementation to psychological development without the mediation of detectable fetal or brain growth.

Still, this possibility, which has come to pass, we saw as remote. We certainly did not anticipate that some of our psychological measures of development would be entirely independent of the more usual measures, and yet be meaningful. Norms for some measures, notably the Bayley tests, were reasonably well established. At the outset, to secure reliable standardized measures, we drew both on Bayley's own work and on the then unpublished experience with the Bayley tests of the large multicenter Collaborative Perinatal Project. The other tests were untried on large or general populations and therefore were not well standardized. Thus, in an array of tests we were gratified to find strong relationships to each other as well as to fetal and infant growth, since the findings reinforced the validity of the tests. We term these measures "growth related." It was a surprise, however, that effects of high protein supplementation were found solely on tests

---

*If we take account of statistically nonsignificant effects, the balanced protein/calorie supplement did better than the high protein supplement, and certainly produced no adverse effects.

quite unrelated either to this interrelated battery of tests or to infant growth. We term these "protein related."

We have advanced reason enough for expecting controversy. Some other choices that we have made in publishing this material deserve mention. Only the results relating most directly to the central hypothesis of the study are reported in this book. A great body of data collateral to the central hypothesis was collected, and a good deal of the data not included here have been analyzed. These analyses are available in three doctoral theses, and in the final report submitted to the National Institute of Child Health and Development. (A bibliography of the study is given in an appendix.)

Certain of the data given in appendices but not discussed in the text bear on the validity of the results and on intervening processes. These include various investigations of the placenta, in particular biochemical measures of cell number and size, the histomorphometry of placental tissue, and the histopathology of the placentae (Appendices 6–8). Their complete analysis and elaboration must await the necessary resources and opportunity. To our generous collaborators Myron Winick and Pedro Rosso, Richard Naeye, and William Blanc, who each directed aspects of this work, we owe apologies for not being able to bring it to completion in this volume.

About these data we can make a number of assertions. We can say that the analysis of the biochemical measures of the placentae (DNA, RNA, and RNase), from which indices of cell number and cell size are derived, do not alter the overall results of the study. In general, we found that these measures added no information over and above that yielded by total placental weight [Pereira, 1977]. Placental weight, in turn, added little information over and above that yielded by birthweight.* Biochemical measures did suggest that the nutritional supplements had an influence on metabolic pathways in the growth process not detectable by the gross measures of outcome devised for the central hypotheses. When analyzed within

---

*One exception relates to maternal smoking: Birthweight was reduced with smoking. Placental weight was not reduced and was therefore greater relative to birthweight than with births of nonsmoking mothers.

treatment groups (and not between treatment groups in
the form the experiment was designed to test) balanced protein/calorie supplementation seemed to have a facilitating
effect on the use of nutrients. This effect may underlie some
outcomes otherwise difficult to explain, for instance, the
absence of maternal weight gain in response to the balanced
protein/calorie supplement. In contrast, with the high protein
supplement, where no similar metabolic processes appeared
to occur, there *was* a response of maternal weight gain to
supplementation.

Histological measures of placental cells and vessels likewise
showed no direct treatment effects. The few significant associations that were found, among many tested, fell into no coherent
pattern, and chance association could not be ruled out. The
data on the pathology of the placenta also seem unlikely to
affect the results relating to the central hypotheses.

This study proved to be a long and arduous undertaking.
The data, the analyses, and the interpretations in this book are
a distillation from huge volumes of material collected over several years and worked into shape over several more years. The
study was conceived early in 1967, funded in mid-1969, and
launched into the field in December 1970. Recruitment of
more than 1,200 eligible women continued over a period of
almost three years, ending in September 1973. The last child
scheduled for a one-year-old examination was seen in the
spring of 1975.

In 1975 and 1976 a further special follow-up of a sample
of study births selected for either premature delivery, low
birthweight, or both, was completed. Prematurely born children had been at risk from adverse effects through gestation
and the perinatal period. The follow-up aimed to discover if
such effects persisted. That selective follow-up is not reported
here, but it brought no results that would cause us to revise
our interpretation of the data up to one year of age. From our
point of view and that of our readers, the important finding
is the absence of detectable ill effects (at two to four years
of age) in the children exposed to the high protein supplement.

This study belongs to a generation of studies of prenatal
nutrition begun in the 1960s that were experimental or quasi-

experimental. As far as physical growth and development are concerned, our study together with others probably marks the end of an era which can be content with gross physical measures of outcome. What can rewardingly be done in that regard has probably been done.

As far as psychological development is concerned, it remains to be seen whether the results reported here are of real significance. If they are, the study could mark the beginning rather than the end of an era. We have found subtle effects on psychological functioning at one year of age that are coherent with other data. We are as yet ignorant about the relationships of such effects to further development. The effects might be too subtle to matter much. On the other hand, mental function being the human phenomenon of ultimate complexity, changes of the kind shown could matter a great deal.

The content of the book can be briefly stated. The first chapter is devoted to a short statement of the rationale of the study, a detailed description of its design, and an account of the processes of recruitment of subjects and their retention in the project. In this chapter we aim to display the scientific foundations of the experiment, and our plans for addressing the pitfalls and snares inherent in studies of the nutrition of free-living human populations.

The second chapter tackles the question, left unanswered in many epidemiological studies and program evaluations, of the effectiveness of the experimental input. Whether or not the nutritional supplementation was used by its intended consumers is crucial to the interpretation of the study. We ask, in effect, whether the experiment took place. While the issue may remain a point of debate, we judge the point well-proved within the limits of available techniques and methods. We have deployed a larger body of indices and analyses than in any other study of this kind known to us. These sustain a conclusion that the nutritional intervention succeeded as well as we could have hoped.

The third chapter outlines the outcome of nutritional intervention in the infants at birth — the crux of the results — and the fourth chapter, the outcome at around one year of age. In these two chapters, as well as in the second chapter, we have provided a quantity of data we judged sufficient to allow readers to satisfy themselves on important points, and yet within the limits of tolerance of our publisher, who has been generous and forbearing.

The fifth chapter gives an overview of the crop of experimental studies of prenatal nutrition of the past decade. We had made a beginning in a recently published paper, and have here developed that conspectus to include outcomes after birth as well as those at birth. In addition, as noted above, in several appendices we have set out analyses of effects of supplementation on an array of placental measures. These appendices are published without comment, for the benefit of the close reader or fellow researcher.

Particular mention should be made of the co-authorship of these appendices and also of Chapters I and IV, which is indicated in the table of contents. This accords inadequate recognition to distinguished colleagues who made important contributions: William Blanc and his colleagues in pediatric pathology at Columbia University; Nathan Brody and his graduate students in psychology at the New School for Social Research; Joseph Fleiss in the Division of Biostatistics of the Columbia University School of Public Health; Richard Naeye and his team at the Department of Pathology at Pennsylvania State University in Hershey, Pennsylvania.

A further note on collegiality is needed. David Rush has given the major part of his research career to this project. Out of concern for the gross disparities in reproductive outcome and child development among social classes in the United States, he had in the mid-sixties begun to plan for a similar project after reviewing the literature and concluding that the way forward lay through a nutritional trial. Out of similar concerns, Zena Stein and I (who have shared ideas, research, and much else for three decades and more) had independently reached the same conclusion. When we obtained the funds to carry out this project, we approached David Rush to join us as its director. We were aware only of his abilities and interests in epidemiology and social pediatrics. The happy coincidence of his particular line of throught with ours brought his ready consent. The outcome, which the reader can judge for himself, is in this book.

Mervyn Susser

Acknowledgments

We wish to make known our indebtedness and gratitude to staff, co-investigators, and participants in the community. In a project first funded in 1969, not all can be mentioned by name. Staff members active virtually throughout the project were Hillard Davis (statistician), Floyd McCormick (field director), Dorothy Jones (administrative secretary), and Albert Nelson (stockman/deliveryman). We must make particular mention, without in any way slighting the contributions of others, of the following: Lillian Belmont for her help with developing psychological measures; Myron Winick, Pedro Rosso, and Mary Campbell Brown for biochemical analyses of the placentae; Richard Naeye for histomorphometry of the placentae; William Blanc, Prem Chauhan, and Carlos Navarro for pathology of the placentae; Donald Swartz for unfailing support in providing access to the obstetric service under his direction; Eric Kahn and Leonard Glass for access to and help with the newborn under their care; George Christakis for early contributions on nutritional questions; Richard Koenigsberger for modifying his neurological examination of the newborn to be used by Project nurses; and, Morton Soifer, Robert Harkins, and Duane Benton who brought the resources of Ross Laboratories to bear in preparing the food supplements. Herman Baker carried out the biochemical tests of maternal serum and urine with great efficiency and the late Francis Marolla made invaluable statistical and design contributions from the earliest stages of the project; Hugh Evans carried out routine testing of cord blood for immunoglobulins and John Sever tested for specific antibodies as the occasion arose. The project was funded under contract No. 1-HD-92190, and was given substantial additional support by the New York State Psychiatric Institute Epidemiology of Mental Retardation Research Unit (Director, Dr. Zena Stein). We also owe much to the tenacious support of Dr. Michael Begab, our Project Officer at the National Institute of Health and Human Development, and to timely advice from Dr. Samuel Greenhouse, then of the same Institute.

Participating Investigators

Principal Investigator:	Mervyn Susser	Gertrude H. Sergievsky Professor of Epidemiology, and Director, Gertrude H. Sergievsky Center, Columbia University
Director of the Project:	David Rush	Associate Professor of Public Health (Epidemiology) and Pediatrics, Columbia University
Co-Investigators:		
Epidemiology:	Zena Stein	Director, Epidemiology of Brain Disorders Research Department, New York Psychiatric Institute, and Professor of Public Health (Epidemiology), Sergievsky Center, Columbia University
Nutrition/Biochemsitry:	Myron Winick	Robert R. Williams Professor of Nutrition and Professor of Pediatrics, and Director, Institute of Human Nutrition, Columbia University
	George Christakis	Professor of Epidemiology and Public Health, University of Miami School of Medicine (formerly Professor of Community Medicine, Mt. Sinai School of Medicine)
Obstetrics:	Donald Swartz	Professor and Chairman of Obstetrics and Gynecology, Albany Medical Center (formerly Professor of Obstetrics and Gynecology, Columbia University)
Pathology:	William Blanc	Professor of Pathology, and Head, Division of Developmental Pathology, College of Physicians and Surgeons, Columbia University

	Richard Naeye	Professor and Chairman, Department of Pathology, Milton S. Hershey Medical Center, Pennsylvania State University College of Medicine
Psychology:	Nathan Brody	Professor and Chairman, Psychology Department, Wesleyan Univeristy (formerly Professor of Psychology, New School for Social Research)
Statistics:	Joseph Fleiss	Professor and Head, Division of Biostatistics, Columbia University School of Public Health
Virology/Immunology:	John Sever	National Institute of Neurology and Communicative Disorders, Bethesda, Maryland
	Hugh Evans	Director of Pediatrics Jewish Hospital Medical Center of Brooklyn (formerly Associate Professor of Pediatrics, Columbia University)

Project Staff

Field Director:	Floyd McCormick
Statistician:	Hillard Davis
Nurses:	Anita Jones Sheila Jozak Linda Kaplan Sybil Patrick Arlene Wilson
Nutritionists:	Ruth Carol Ruby Dickens Charlotte Duncan Dahlia Gordon Lorelei Sarli
Computer Programmer:	Hillel Cohen
Psychologists:	Karen Dorros Alice Edelman Judith Feldman Alan Gottfried

Edith Jacobs
Daniel Johnson
John Kiely
Raphel Lakowitz
Janet Marcus
Thelma Markowitz
Stephen Salay
Patricia Singleton
Guido Zanni, Jr.

Health Aides: Sarah Benbow
Audrey Brown
Lila Brown
Audrey Cameron
Loraine Fulgham
Pearline Green
Alma Hill
Louise Lowery
Verline Quick
Josephine Shields

Stockmen/Deliverymen: Leonard Ingram
Albert Nelson

Statistical Clerks: Alice Abadin
Carol Studemire

Laboratory Technicians: Phyllis Alexander
Miriam Paige

Secretaries: Mary Hendricks
Wendy Hulen
Sandra Pond
Jane Reeves
Ann Wallace
Juliet Williams

Research Assistants: Patricia Crawford
Mary Leahey
Patricia Zybert

Clerk/Chaperones: Bruce Dean
James Harding

Graduate Research Assistants: Barbara Mayleas
Mandhana Nuchpakdee
Mauricio Pereira
Carol Wilkinson

Administrative Secretaries: Alice Hoffer
Dorothy Jones

Chapter I

Rationale and Design of the Study, and Enrollment of the Sample*

RATIONALE

Disparities in perinatal mortality and child development are marked between American whites and blacks, and between children of high and low social status. A manifest public health need is to discover environmental causes of such disparities, and find ways to reverse them. This study, a main strut of a program so directed, sought an effective means of intervention. It was funded in 1969, and was conducted in parallel with a study of the effects of prenatal nutritional deprivation during the Dutch famine of 1944–45 [Stein et al, 1975].

We have shown elsewhere that birthweight could account for the whole of the twofold excess in the perinatal mortality of blacks over whites in New York City and in Rochester [Bergner and Susser, 1970; Rush, 1972]. Length of gestation, including premature deliveries and postmature deliveries, contributed relatively little to perinatal mortality independently of birthweight [Susser, Marolla, and Fleiss, 1972]. Many writers [Drillien, 1972; Neligan et al, 1976; Pasamanick and Knobloch, 1966; Wiener et al, 1968], if not all [Douglas, 1960; McKeown, 1970], have held birthweight also to be an important predictor of subsequent development and handicap, especially in interaction with adverse postnatal environment [Birch and Gussow, 1970]. We concluded that fetal growth was likely to be an intervening process of importance to the course of subsequent development.

Since nutrition is essential to growth, it has long seemed plausible that maternal nutrition is crucial to fetal growth. In a review of the literature relating maternal nutrition to birthweight [Bergner and Susser, 1970], we advocated a randomized, controlled trial of nutritional supplementation in pregnancy, with the aim of raising mean birthweight and influencing later development.

*Joseph Fleiss is a co-author of this chapter.

Previous experimental studies of the effect of maternal dietary supplementation on birthweight were inconclusive, and none had followed later development. Conflict and confusion among the results of previous studies could be attributed to flaws in design, execution, and analysis. A well-designed, well-executed experimental intervention seemed to offer the best hope for obtaining a definitive answer. Our review of the evidence showed that environmental manipulation was a rational approach. The factors that influenced birthweight within racially homogenous populations were preeminently environmental and not genetic. These factors related to the wider environment of the mother, for example social and economic status; to the mother's own growth and nutrition, for example height, preconception weight, and weight gain during pregnancy; and to the mother's behavior, for example smoking.

We also confirmed that maternal prepregnant weight and weight gain during pregnancy could be seen as a final common pathway of the well-known associations between birthweight and maternal age, height, and parity [Rush, Davis, and Susser, 1972; Stein et al, 1975]. Certainly maternal nutrient intake influences maternal weight and weight gain. Weight gain during pregnancy pointed to processes current during the gestation of the affected infant, and focused attention on the present state of the mother, rather than on previous experience during her own growth [Bergner and Susser, 1970].

The hope that fetal growth was accessible to intervention during gestation was encouraged by the further conclusion that the variation in birthweight owed to environmental forces was a consequence of variation in fetal growth in the third trimester of pregnancy [Bergner and Susser, 1970]. The effects of the Dutch famine on the birthweight of successive cohorts exposed at different stages of gestation [Stein et al, 1975] lent striking support to comparisons of birthweight by gestational age among singleton and multiple births [McKeown and Record, 1953], as well as to comparisons among different populations [Gruenwald, 1966]. All these pointed to third trimester variation. It seemed, therefore, that we need not be deterred by the difficulties that were likely to be encountered in engaging women at high risk of low birthweight and in the first thirty weeks of pregnancy in a program of nutritional supplementation.

Observational studies had yielded some answers to the questions at issue under the extreme conditions of famine, but uncertain answers under the ordinary conditions of daily life, especially in populations without evidence of clinical malnutrition. Most observational studies stumble over two major weaknesses. First, available techniques for determining nutritional intake and energy expenditure in free-living populations suffer from a notable lack of precision. Second, many facets of poverty that are linked with retarded growth and development are also closely associated with poor nutrition, and thereby potentially confound the relation of nutrition with growth and development.

Two major observational studies of the 1950s had been taken as evidence against the hypothesis that maternal nutrition influenced birthweight. Thomson [1959] in Aberdeen, Scotland, had found a significant association between maternal calorie intake during pregnancy and birthweight, but discounted this result; he considered that the association was explained by maternal size, an antecedent common to both calorie intake and birthweight. Against Thomson we argued that his analysis did not in fact eliminate, nor indeed test, the alternative hypothesis that caloric intake influenced birthweight, and that his interpretation was therefore too restrictive. Darby et al [1953] in Nashville, Tennessee, found only one tenuous relationship of maternal nutrient intake with birthweight. Vitamin C alone, of many nutrients analyzed, had a significant association. Against the conclusion that maternal nutrition did not influence birthweight, one could argue that the weakness of the measures of nutrient intake could suppress a significant association. Equally telling, in the populations under observation low birthweight was infrequent; they may therefore not have been above the threshold where nutritional variation would have much effect. On these grounds, we decided that a new experimental study was justified. Our funding agency — the National Institute of Child Health and Human Development, Mental Retardation Branch — agreed, and we were able to proceed.

In succeeding chapters, we shall report first on the design and method of the study; second, on the extent to which the experimental intervention actually took place; third, on outcomes at birth for the entire study group; and fourth, on outcomes in the offspring at approximately one year of age. Finally, we place the results of this study in the context of other contemporary studies of prenatal nutrition in free-living populations.

DESIGN

Among several outcome measures, birthweight was chosen as the critical dependent variable around which sample size was determined. Birthweight is measured easily, routinely, and with high reliability. Also, experience with birthweight exceeds that with any other index of fetal growth in both clinical and epidemiologic study. The birthweight index was supplemented by several measures of fetal growth and developmental outcome. Gestational age was included among these both as an outcome, and as a control variable necessary to the assessment of fetal growth.

The independent study variable was the level of nutritional supplementation during pregnancy, determined by assignment to one of three treatment groups. One group was assigned to a high protein supplement, a second to a balanced supplement with much lower content of protein and fewer calories, and a third to routine clinic supplements without any additions. Random assignment and stratification by a number of potentially confounding variables before assignment, were used to achieve comparability among the groups. Comparability was judged from the distribution of attributes of the women across treatment groups. The population was stratified on three variables known to be highly associated with birthweight (prepregnancy weight, weight gain during pregnancy, history of having borne an infant of low birthweight). Since the effect of protein intake on birthweight was a central question in this study, the population was also stratified on a measure of protein intake. All results were analyzed by comparing the means of the outcome measures, as well as by multivariate techniques to control for confounding and to discover the presence and extent of suppression or distortion [Susser, 1973].

Sample Size

In New York City at the outset of the study, birthweight among blacks was about 125 gm lower than among whites. An increase of 125 gm in mean birthweight of blacks would have virtually eliminated the almost two-fold difference referred to above between the current black and white perinatal mortality, assuming constant birthweight-specific mortality rates [Bergner and Susser, 1970; Rush, 1972]. A sample size was therefore chosen such that a mean difference between experimental and control groups of 125 gm in weight at birth would be expected to occur by chance no more than 5% of the time by two-tailed test ($\alpha = 0.05$), and the difference would be detected 80% of the time ($\beta = 0.2$).

On this basis, the required size of each treatment group was about 250. With three treatment groups we needed to ensure that 750 women continued the treatment regimen up to the time of delivery of a singleton birth. We allowed for a 25% loss from initial recruitment up to the time of delivery. In fact, of the 1,051 women recruited into the study, 770 remained participants up to delivery and gave birth to living singleton infants. The smallest of the three groups included 249 liveborn singletons.

Target Population and Selection Criteria

The target population was selected from the clinic of a municipal hospital serving mainly the indigent of a large black community in New York City. At the initiation of the study, the proportion of infants in this hospital weighing under 2,500 gm at birth was about 18%, three times that of the more affluent areas of the city. The perinatal mortality rate of the area in question (72/1,000 in 1965) had been generally about double that of the city as a whole. Because protein-rich foods are expensive, and because past surveys indicated strong gradients of protein intake with socioeconomic status, we expected to find low levels of protein intake. Information gathered in preparation for the study about the nutritional state of pregnant women in the target population and other similar groups supported this view.

Certain women were excluded from the trial. Thus, women were not asked to participate if they were known to be seeking an abortion, if they had specific chronic health disorders (eg cardiac disease, diabetes, hypertension, or chronic kidney disease, including recurrent urinary tract infection), or if they admitted to recent use of narcotics or heavy use of alcohol. In order to be eligible, women had to be black, English-speaking, and not further advanced than 30 weeks gestation at interview.

We selected the target population on the grounds that the lower the expected birthweight, the greater the likelihood that improved diet would increase it. Therefore, we set criteria for participation that would select women whose risk of bearing infants of low birthweight was above average for this community. These criteria were also meant to be coherent with a nutritional etiology for low birthweight.

The criteria were arrived at after preliminary work on nearly 10,000 recent maternities in the hospital that was to be the site of the controlled trial [Rush, Davis, and Susser, 1972]. Three years of computerized records coded for birthweight, length of gestation, and a number of maternal attributes were available for the study. Among the coded attributes which were known to carry a high risk for low birthweight were maternal age, parity, height, prepregnant weight, weight gain during pregnancy, and history of previous low birthweight delivery. All these associations were confirmed in the data.

Further multivariate analysis led to a consolidation of these risk criteria and, consequently, to a reduction in their number and a simplification of the research design. We were able to show that the associations with low birthweight of maternal age, parity and height were entirely accounted for by prepregnant weight and weight gain during pregnancy. Only history of previous low birthweight was not accounted for by these two factors, which together comprise maternal weight.

Rationale and Design of the Study / 7

As noted above, we had previously argued that the associations of low birthweight with maternal weight supported the hypothesis that maternal nutrition influenced birthweight. Our multivariate analysis now allowed us to develop a causal model coherent for a number of these factors, as follows:

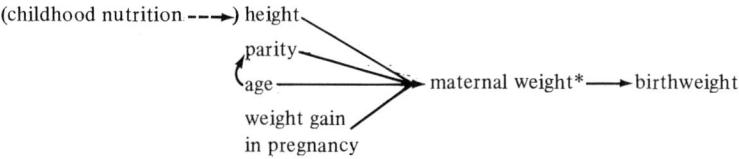

*Maternal weight = prepregnant weight + weight gain.

This model can be elaborated in the following manner to include the untested causal paths (shown in broken lines) that are the subject of the present study:

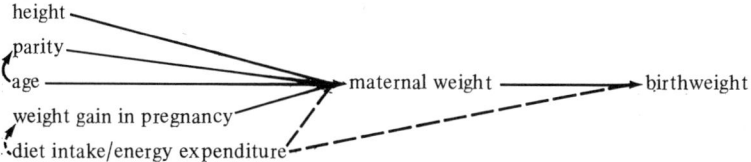

This model permitted the rational choice of two known high-risk factors for low birthweight (weight gain in pregnancy and maternal weight) and a third hypothetical one (diet intake), as selection criteria for high risk appropriate to a nutritional study. We decided also to use previous history of low birthweight as a selection criterion for high risk. Although the mechanism involved was obscure to us, within the categories of prepregnant weight and weight gain in pregnancy this factor did contribute independently to birthweight.

In accord with these ideas, only women who weighed less than 140 lbs (63 kg) at conception were recruited. Before assigning a woman randomly to a treatment group, we first ascertained that she fulfilled at least one of the following additional criteria:

    1) Low prepregnant weight (under 110 pounds [50 kg] at conception): in this group we expected, from prior experience at this hosptial, that the mean birthweight for term deliveries (37 weeks) would be about 2,900 gm.

2) Low weight gain up to the time of recruitment: in this group, we estimated, from expected weight gain projected from the initial weight gain, that the mean birthweight for term deliveries would be about 2,850 gm.

3) At least one previous low birthweight infant: in this group we expected that the mean birthweight for term deliveries would be about 2,720 gm.

4) A history of protein intake less than 50 gm in the 24 hours preceding registration, as calculated by the nutritionist from a 24-hour quantitative dietary recall. There were no data allowing us to predict the average birthweight in this group, but the criterion was chosen for its coherence with our hypothesis. From prior study we expected that, as a group, women selected by this criterion would have a consistently lower mean protein intake than the average woman using this hospital.

We used these selection criteria as attributes on which to stratify the study population before randomization for two reasons. One reason, noted above, was to ensure an equal distribution of these attributes across treatment groups, and thereby control confounding. The second reason was to define conditions under which women might differ in their responses to treatment, and hence to differentiate them in the experimental framework. The groups were formed by taking all combinations of the following characteristics: 1) low maternal weight at conception and/or low weight gain from conception to recruitment*; 2) past history of bearing a low ($<$ 2,500 gm) birthweight infant; 3) history of protein intake of under 50 gm in the 24 hours before registration.

Cigarette smoking was also known to have a substantial effect on birthweight and to be frequent enough in the population to cause confounding. At that time, we did not conceive of smoking as a possible conditional variable that might alter

---

*The criterion for low weight gain was read off a table of values of weight gain prepared from data on the clinic population before the beginning of recruitment to the study proper.

the relation between nutrition and birthweight.* We decided therefore to rely on random assignment and analysis to control confounding, in order not to overcomplicate the process of stratifying.

To preserve the comparability of the treatment groups, procedures for replacing women who dropped out of the study were developed. Initially, when a woman was unable to complete the study regimen, the next woman who appeared and met the criteria of the same recruitment category was assigned to her treatment group. By this means we tried to ensure that each treatment group would not only be of sufficient size for an adequate test of the hypothesis (allowed for in the 25% estimated attrition rate), but that each group would have the same distribution of stratifying criteria at the end of the study. We stopped this nonrandom replacement procedure after the first 48 replacements. In practice, the stratification categories of women dropping out differed little among the treatment groups, and replacement was difficult to achieve because it interfered with the routine assignment procedure. Throughout, we collected all available information on perinatal outcome among women who dropped out to enable us to judge the effect of selective loss of subjects on the final results.

Forms of Treatment

Nutritional supplementation was supplied in the form of two different beverages (Table 1.1).** As noted, one beverage provided a high protein supplement and the other a balanced calorie/protein supplement with a lower total calorie content. Both beverages supplied additional minerals and vitamins, and an especially high level of riboflavin. Although

---

*In the light of subsequent research, including the results of this study, smoking does appear to be a conditional variable that interacts with nutritional state to affect birthweight [Rush, 1974; Davies et al, 1976].

**We are indebted to Ross Laboratories for development and manufacturing of these supplements.

TABLE 1.1. Composition of Daily Diet Supplements for Each Treatment Group

Component	Treatment group		
	Supplement	Complement	Controls
Protein (casein) (gm)	40.0	6.0	–
Carbohydrate (gm)	55.0	57.4	–
Fat (gm)	8.6	7.6	–
Calories	470.0	322.0	–
Calcium (mg)	1,000.0	250.0	250.0
Magnesium (mg)	100.0	12.0	0.15
Iron[a] (mg)	60.0	40.0	117
Zinc (mg)	4.0	0.084	0.085
Copper (mg)	2.0	0.15	0.15
Iodine (μg)	150.0	100.0	100.0
Vitamin A (IU)	6,000.0	4,000.0	4,000.0
Vitamin D (IU)	400.0	400.0	400.0
Vitamin E (USPU)	30	–	–
Vitamin C (mg)	60.0	60.0	60.0
Vitamin B_1 (mg)	3.0	3.0	3.0
Vitamin B_2 (mg)	15.0	15.0	2.0
Niacin (mg)	15.0	10.0	10.0
Vitamin B_6 (mg)	2.5	3.0	3.0
Pantothenic acid (mg)	1.0	1.0	1.0
Biotin (μg)	200	not analyzed	–
Folic acid (μg)	350.0	350.0	350.0
Vitamin B_{12} (μg)	8.0	3.0	3.0
Volume	16 ounces	16 ounces	1 capsule

[a]Elemental iron (78 mg) prescribed for all patients on beverage in addition to beverage.

the beverages were specifically prepared processed foods and unlike foods in the regular diet, their use conferred several advantages on an experimental study. The nutrient composition of the supplements was known with precision. They allowed for double-blinded study between the two supplemented groups because the cans which contained the beverages could be identical in appearance. The amounts drunk were amenable to better recall and measurement than the regular diet. Actual use of the supplements could be monitored by measuring the excretion rate of the riboflavin included in excess in both beverages. Finally, they could be prescribed in the manner of a medication specifically intended for pregnancy. By characterizing the supplements as special to pregnancy, we aimed to minimize the dispersion of the products by the recipients to others than themselves. The women were repeatedly advised to take beverages as supplements to the regular diet, and not as replacements for it.

On the other hand, the use of foods that were not part of an everyday diet created uncertainty for the project since we could not be sure of their acceptability. Before the pilot study, trials to judge the palatability and acceptability of the beverage were performed with a population drawn from a clinic similar to that selected for the study. We then tested all procedures in a pilot study in the same clinic as that used in the definitive study. In both these trials, the beverages proved acceptable.

The three study groups received one of the following treatments (Table 1.1):

Supplement: Two 8-ounce cans of beverage daily, that provided a daily total of 40 gm of animal protein, 470 calories, and an array of vitamins and minerals. There was a choice of three flavors (chocolate, vanilla, cherry).

Complement: Two 8-ounce cans of beverage daily, packaged identically with the same flavors as Supplement, that provided a daily total of 6 gm of animal protein, 322 calories, and the same amount of vitamins and minerals as were in the prenatal tablet used in the clinic.

Control (nonintervention group): Continuation of regular clinic care, including standard multivitamin/mineral tablets.

Apart from the major difference in protein content, there were minor differences in other nutrients between Supplement and Complement (Table 1.1). Among these, only zinc has been suggested as possibly important to fetal development, and the amount of zinc in Supplement is typical of the zinc content of naturally occurring high protein foods. Because of these minor differences in other nutrients, effects perceived as due to protein cannot be entirely separated from effects of these others, but the likelihood of confounding is remote. It is therefore the high protein content of Supplement that should differentiate its effects from those of Complement. At the initiation of this study, lack of protein was generally viewed as the deficiency among the poor most likely to endanger development. Surveys had indicated that protein intake decreased with declining social status, and animal experiments had shown that severe protein deprivation could limit brain growth [Winick and Noble, 1966; Zamenhof, van Marthens, and Margolis, 1968]. The degree of protein deprivation in the target population was not presumed to compare in degree with that in these animal experiments. Yet there seemed good reason for postulating a continuous dose-response effect, with protein as the most likely critical limiting nutrient.*

The high protein Supplement and the balanced protein and calorie Complement treatment groups were exposed to identical experiences in the study, apart from the differences in composition between the beverages. Both groups were encouraged and instructed in the regular use of beverages. The flavoring was the same for both, and the cans bore identical labels. Excepting the statistics staff, neither participants nor other staff were aware which of the two beverages was being supplied. Women receiving beverages were also given 78 mg elemental iron daily, separately from the beverage, to adjust their intake to the 117 mg daily that was routinely prescribed by the clinic. The monitoring of food and beverage intake, and the regular field and clinic contact and support, were the same for both groups. As a device for monitoring the intake of the beverages, each can contained 7.5 mg of riboflavin. This level was considered harmless by all experts consulted. Although within the therapeutic range, the amount was enough to allow measurement of excess riboflavin excreted in the urine.

Although beverage use was double-blind, the women in the Control group were necessarily made aware, by our procedure of obtaining informed consent prior to random treatment group assignment, that they did not receive supplements while other women did. Thus, responses to the form rather

---

*Several years later, we convinced ourselves in our study of the Dutch famine that the effect of severe nutritional deprivation was not linear and continuous, but only became manifest below a threshold value [Stein et al, 1975]. We also learned from the Guatemala intervention study [Habicht et al, 1974] that calories might be the most important nutritional constituent in accelerating fetal growth in an undernourished population.

than to the content of the treatment could not be neutralized as between the Control group and the two supplemented groups. We attempted as far as possible to shield the project staff who assessed outcome from knowledge of whether or not a participant had received beverage supplements. Since maternal weight gain, duration of gestation, and birthweight were taken from clinic and hospital records, the likelihood that assessments of these outcomes were biased by knowledge of treatment group assignment is virtually nil.

The first function of the Control group was to represent norms for comparison, against which deviations from regular diet and changes in birthweight among the two supplemented treatment groups could be detected. With regard to birthweight, the detection of a dose-response gradient or other patterns across the three experimental groups could be equally important for inference and interpretation.

A second function of the nonsupplemented Control group was to aid in separating effects of the beverage format itself, and the special attention associated with it, from the intended effects of the contents of the two diet supplements alone. To identify such inadvertent effects of intervention, we relied upon the expectation that nonnutritional effects would be equal in the two beverage-supplemented groups, and absent in the nonsupplemented Control group. By contrast, our expectation was that the intended nutritional effects would occur unequally in a graded pattern across the three treatment groups. An effect owed solely to the protein increment should show a clear advantage for the Supplement group over both the Complement and nonsupplemented Control groups. An effect owed to calories should show a gradient running from the Supplement, through the Complement, to the Control group.

Procedures

The flow chart in Figure 1.1 illustrates the procedures followed in the enrollment of the study population. All procedures were tested and the participating personnel were trained in their administration during a pilot experimental period that lasted about six months (following one month's recruitment) before the study proper began.

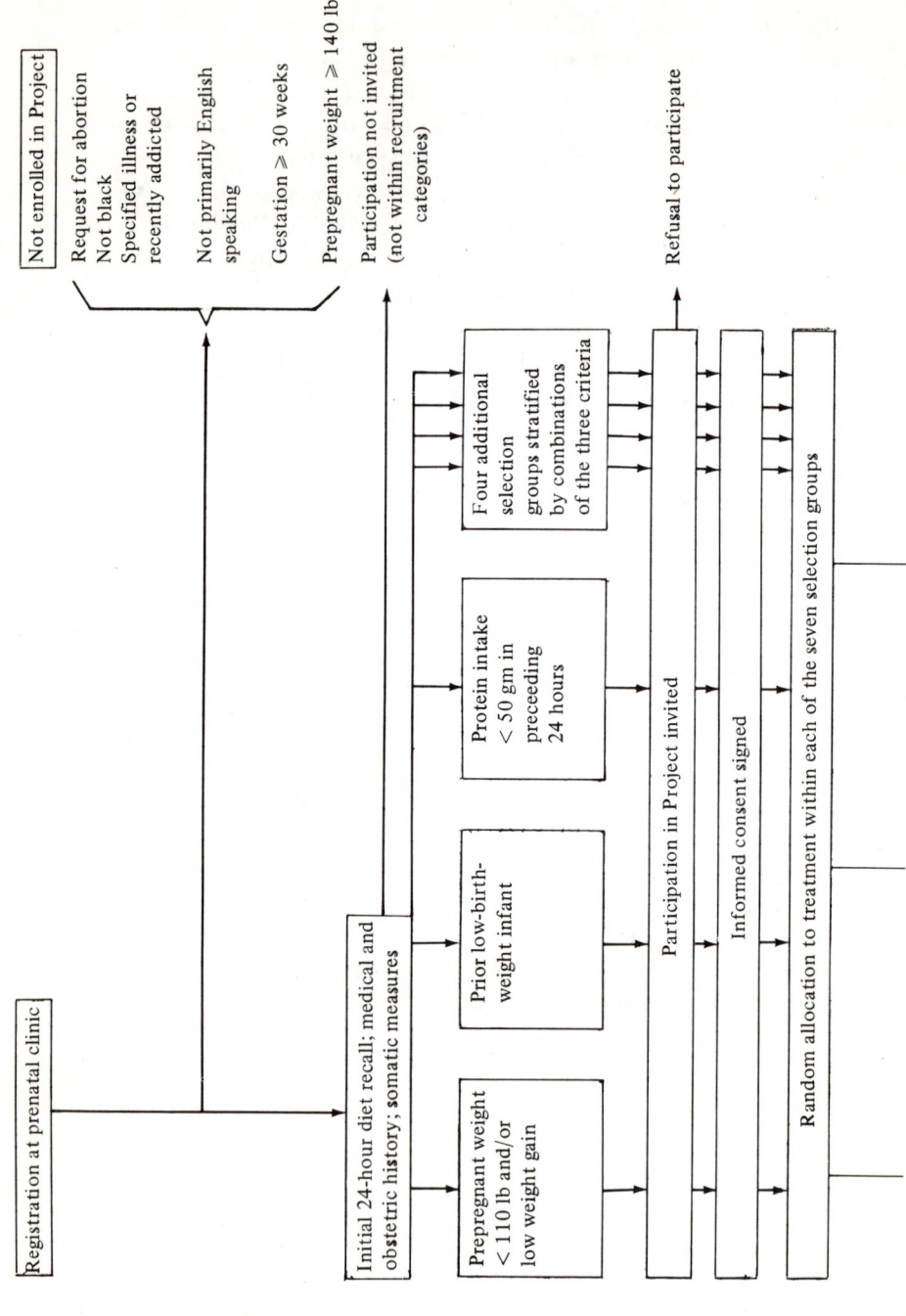

Rationale and Design of the Study / 15

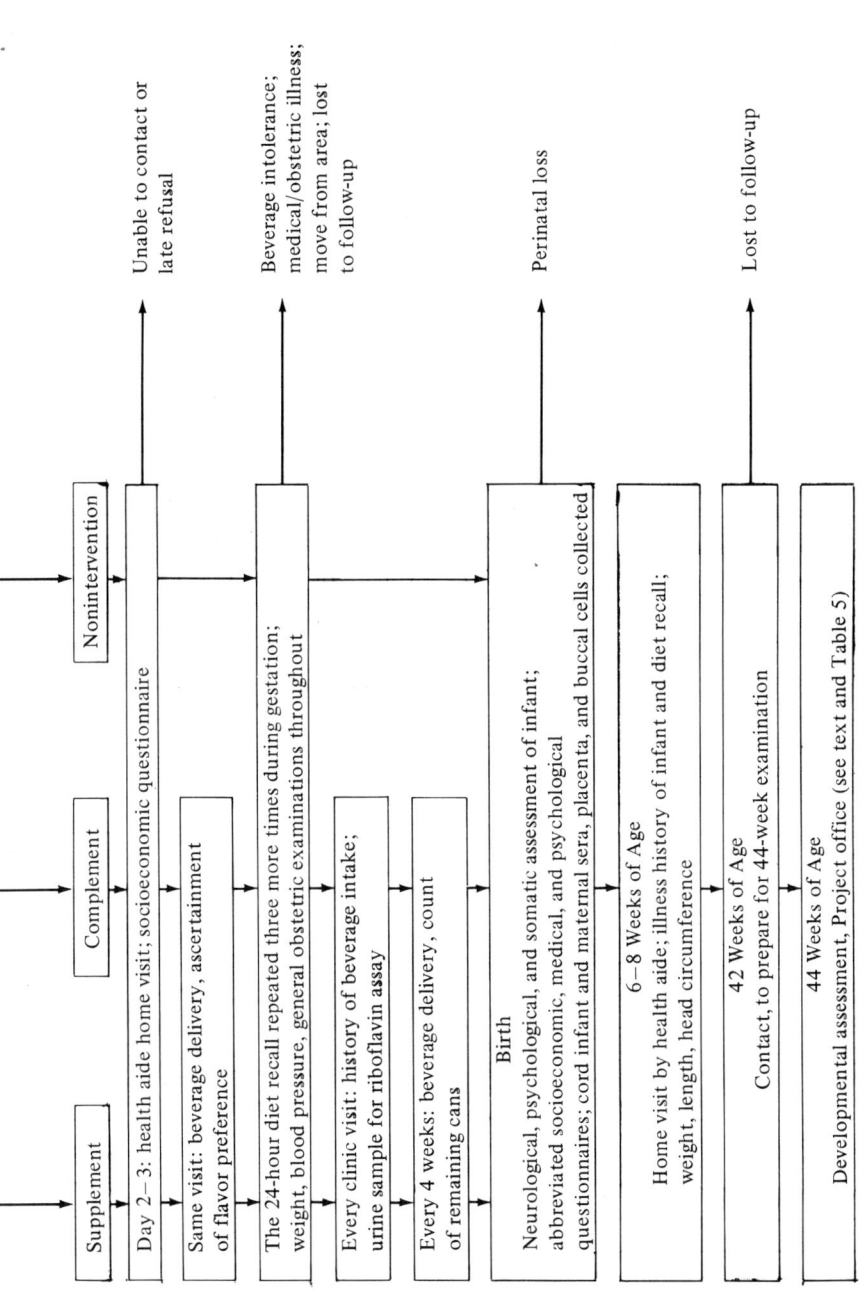

Fig. 1.1. Sequence of procedures for women registering for prenatal care. Taken from Rush et al, 1974.

Appendix 1.1 is a synopsis of the data collected at entry to the study and during the prenatal period, and Appendix 1.2 is a synopsis of the data collected at delivery and at follow-up for the first year after delivery. At each prenatal clinic the project nurse screened every woman registering for her first prenatal visit for eligibility for the study. Next the project nutritionist took a quantitative 24-hour dietary history, in order that low protein intake could be used as a criterion for recruitment and stratification. The project nurse then completed the medical and obstetric history. She weighed each woman and measured height, arm girth, and skinfold thickness. At this point, with screening for eligibility completed and the data for stratification collected, those eligible were invited to participate. The three alternative treatments and the process of random assignment were described to potential participants in some detail. Those who consented in writing to participating in the study were classified within one of the seven strata derived from all the combinations of the stratification criteria. Random assignment to a treatment group followed.

Before a woman was classed as an active participant, she was visited at home within several days by a health aide especially trained and regularly supervised. An extensive social history was taken. If the woman was assigned to a beverage, an initial supply was provided.

During the course of the pregnancy, beverage deliveries were made monthly. At each delivery of beverage, a count of unused cans was made. (This procedure was instituted only about one-third of the way through the study.) At each clinic, the clinic staff weighed all patients, including study participants. The balance was regularly standardized. A health aide took a history of beverage intake from all women receiving a beverage, and she collected a urine specimen to be analyzed for riboflavin level. Twenty-four hour dietary recalls were taken by the study nutritionists a second time at the first return visit two weeks after recruitment, a third time one month after that, and a fourth time close to 32 weeks gestation. Analyses of serum vitamin levels were done on blood routinely collected by the clinic staff at registration and, when possible, at delivery.

A project nurse was informed by the clinical service of the admission of the study participants for delivery. The project nurse repeated an abbreviated social history, and abstracted medical information from the hospital records. The social history served to test reliability on items that should not have changed, but also to discover in other items changes relevant to the study. The baby was weighed at birth by the hospital staff on a balance that was checked regularly by project staff. A specimen of cord blood was obtained. The placenta was put aside for the project nurse to trim, weigh, and take a wedge for freezing and subsequent biochemical analysis. The remainder was prepared for pathological examination according to standard procedures, all within 24 hours of birth, but usually sooner. The project nurse transcribed relevant data on the delivery onto precoded project forms.

Between 48 and 72 hours after delivery, the project nurse weighed the infant, measured its length, head size, arm girth, and skinfold thickness, carried out standard physical and neurological examination (for which she had been specially trained) and assessed habituation to a tactile stimulus. Examinations of infants under special care were deferred. Nurses and psychologists were kept unaware of treatment group assignment and of the recorded date of mother's last menstrual period.

Special efforts were made to trace women who failed to return for clinic visits scheduled in relation to the project. In those few cases where a woman had moved locally, or where she had chosen to be confined in another local hospital (45 in all), birthweight and other relevant information were abstracted from the chart at a later date, but placentas were not collected, nor were newborn examinations made.

Six to eight weeks after delivery, each mother was visited at home. At this visit, the weight and dietary history of the infant was recorded. A brief social history was taken and changes in the family situation noted. After this visit, the project field staff renewed contact with the mother by telephone or mail several weeks before the child's examination at about one year of age fell due. If a mother had moved from the city (about 15% left New York, usually to return to homes in the South), she was offered travel expenses in order to return for the assessment of the infant.

At the assessment at around one year of age, a social history was again taken from the mother as well as a history of the health, development and diet of the infant. Over a period lasting two to three hours, the infant was given a battery of psychological tests by two or three project psychologists under the direction of Dr. Nathan Brody. The infant was also weighed and measured for height, skinfold thickness, and head circumference. Reliability measures were developed among the psychologists.

A number of laboratories were involved in testing specimens collected for the project. One laboratory (Dr. Herman Baker) measured levels of serum vitamins (A, B_6, absorbic acid) and urine riboflavin. Dr. Myron Winick's laboratory made biochemical assays of the placenta; Dr. William Blanc's laboratory examined its gross and microscopic pathology; and Dr. Richard Naeye developed methods for histomorphometry of the placenta. Dr. Hugh Evans measured the immunoglobulin M in the three-day old infant's blood, and in cases of raised IgM, Dr. John Sever tested the cord blood and the mother's sera at registration and delivery for specific antibodies. For each of these tests, a particular procedure was developed to monitor reliability.

Outcome Measures

Birthweight was copied from routine hospital records and validated by our own measurements at two to three days of life. We also abstracted data that dealt with the physiological state of the infant at birth (including the elements that go to make up the Apgar score) as well as the clinical progress on the ward (feeding, temperature, infection and other indices of overall health).

Infant weight, length, head circumference, arm circumference and skinfold thickness (subscapular and triceps) were available from the project nurse's observation between 48 and

72 hours of age. The nurse's examination also afforded indices of newborn maturity; these were derived from the work of Usher, McLean, and Scott [1966] and from a neurological examination prepared and modified by Koenigsberger [1966] as well as tests of laterality and habituation to tactile stimuli. From the psychologist's examinations there were available systematic observations at 72 hours of age on the infant's state and activity level, and also on behavioral organization, habituation to auditory stimuli, and visual pursuit.

The placenta was evaluated for gross and microscopic abnormalities, in terms of histomorphometry, and biochemically for deoxyribonucleic acid (DNA), ribonucleic acid (RNA), protein, and alkaline ribonuclease (RNase). Capillary blood (taken from the routine heel-prick for phenylketonuria [PKU] testing) was screened for raised immunoglobulin levels. Where these were raised, maternal and cord blood were tested for specific antibodies.

RECRUITMENT, SELECTION, ATTRITION

The recruitment process is illustrated in Figure 1.2 and Table 1.2. During the recruitment period, from mid-December 1970 through early September 1973, a total of 6,335 women registered at the prenatal clinic. Of these, 1,255 were deemed eligible and 1,051 women in all agreed to participate. Eight hundred and fourteen participants remained active in the study until delivery. One hundred twenty-one women, after agreeing to participate, did not become active in the study, either because they were belatedly discovered not to have been eligible, or because they could not be found when the initial visit to the home was made, or because they decided not to participate before the visit was completed. Forty-three moved from the New York City area. Fourteen women, of whom half were in the Supplement group, were discontinued in the study for medical reasons. The differences between groups were accounted for by those with diabetes or abnormal glucose tolerance curves (4 in the Supplement group, 2 in the Complement group, and 1 in the Control group). Fifty-nine women discontinued beverage use, 27 in the Supplement group, and 32 in the Complement group.

Numbers of women within each risk stratum who remained active to delivery did not differ much by treatment group (Table 1.2). Nine of 814 women bore twins, unevenly distributed among the treatment groups. Thirty-six fetal deaths, distributed nearly equally among the three treatment groups, depleted the sample at birth. Birthweights were recorded on fewer than half the fetal deaths. No bias in the distribution of outcome variables is anticipated from the omissions of the fetal deaths from analyses of fetal growth: numbers and mean length of gestation of fetal deaths were similar in each treatment group.

At delivery, in the experimental population of 814 women, there were 770 liveborn singletons; one with a major congenital anomaly (Down syndrome) was excluded in further analyses. Fourteen neonatal deaths occurred among these 770 liveborn singletons, and 5 among the 17 liveborn twins.

The distribution of the risk criteria used for the stratification of the experimental population was similar in each treatment group (Table 1.2). The one discrepancy of any note within the several strata was that in the Control group the number with only low prepregnant weight and/or weight gain was smaller, and the number with low prepregnant weight and/or weight gain combined with low protein intake was larger.*

Other Attributes of Treatment Groups

Data on characteristics of all women delivering liveborn singleton infants (omitting the one who delivered an infant diagnosed as having Down syndrome) are shown in Table 1.3. These variables were selected as likely to have meaningful relationships with birthweight and with other perinatal and developmental outcomes.

There were no significant differences among treatment groups for the 12 social and demographic variables. Quetelet's index at conception (weight divided by height squared) was

---

*This difference is controlled in the analyses; it had no effect on any of the outcomes considered in this monograph.

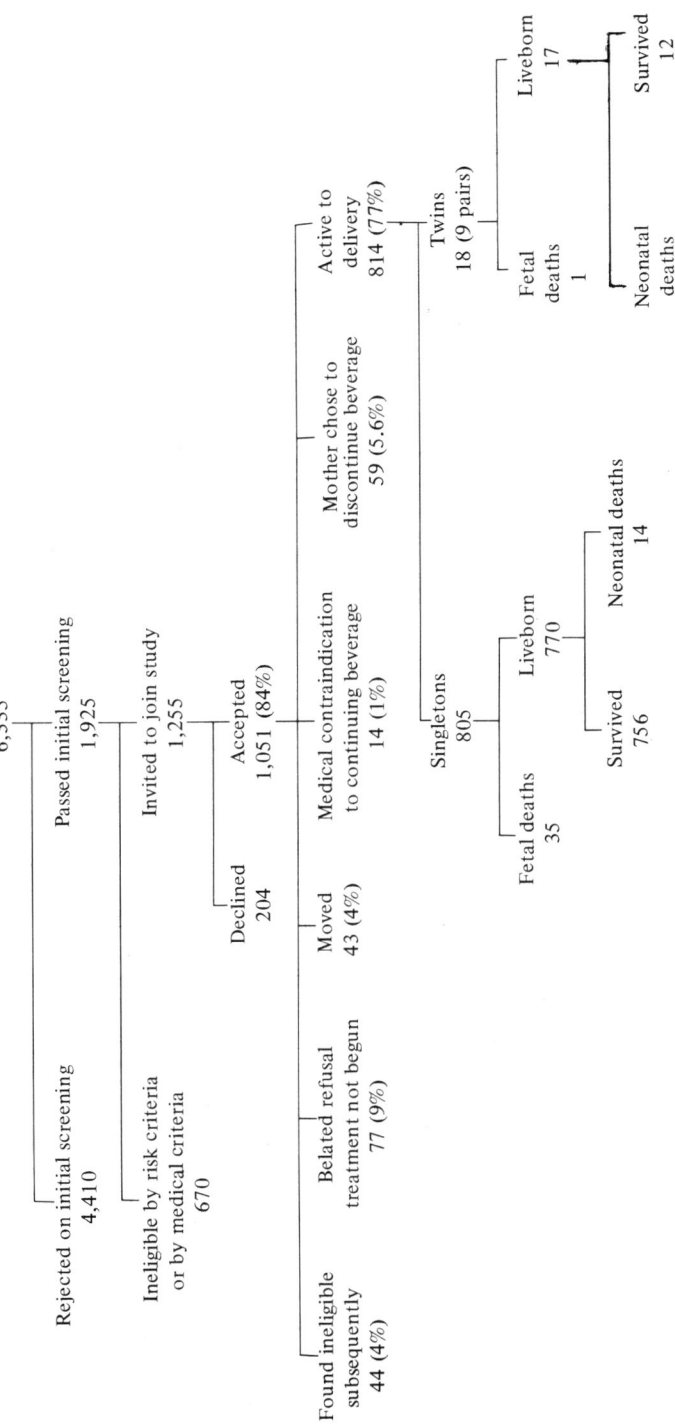

Fig. 1.2. Retention and Attrition. Survival in the study through pregnancy and the newborn period among all women recruited.

TABLE 1.2. Retention and Attrition

Treatment group	(1) Low protein intake only	(2) Past low birthwt only	(3) (1) & (2)	(4) Low wt/wt gain only	(5) (1) & (4)	(6) (2) & (4)	(7) (1) & (2) & (4)	Total
Supplement	55 (6:5)	10 (3:2)	6 (1:0)	117 (30:14)	57 (17:5)	12 (4:1)	6 (4:0)	263 (65:27)
Complement	50 (10:5)	12 (2:1)	8 (0:0)	120 (21:13)	59 (10:12)	14 (3:0)	9 (0:1)	272 (46:32)
Control	53 (11:0)	12 (4:0)	6 (2:0)	114 (36:0)	69 (12:0)	16 (1:0)	9 (1:0)	279 (67:0)
Total	158 (27:10)	34 (9:3)	20 (3:0)	351 (87:27)	185 (39:17)	42 (8:1)	24 (5:1)	814 (178:59)

Number of women who actively continued in study to delivery, by treatment group and strata derived from the three recruitment criteria. (In parentheses: number of belated refusals, moved, medical reasons – before colon; numbers who voluntarily discontinued beverage – after colon).

TABLE 1.3. Characteristics of Study Population

Characteristic	Supplement	Complement	Control
Age (yr)	21.5 ± 4.7	21.9 ± 4.8	21.8 ± 4.7
Primigravidae (%)	54.2	46.5	48.5
Parity[a] (n)	1.9 ± 1.1	1.8 ± 1.2	2.1 ± 1.7
Past low birthweight[a] (n)	0.4 ± 0.9	0.4 ± 0.8	0.4 ± 0.8
Past stillbirth[a] (n)	0.27 ± 0.52	0.30 ± 0.49	0.24 ± 0.51
Past neonatal death[a] (n)	0.061 ± 0.274	0.036 ± 0.188	0.044 ± 0.205
Students (%)	16.5	20.4	17.9
Mothers' education (yr)	10.9 ± 1.6	11.0 ± 1.7	10.8 ± 1.7
Married (%)	26.5	30.1	30.3

Welfare recipient (%)	26.5	24.6	24.6
Foreign born (%)	11.6	10.5	14.4
Southern born[b] (%)	46.4	53.1	52.2
At conception:			
Height (cm)	159.7 ± 6.0	160.2 ± 6.7	159.5 ± 6.3
Weight (lb)	116.2 ± 12.6	115.1 ± 12.3	116.4 ± 13.1
Ponderal index (kg/m^2)	20.67 ± 2.35	20.32* ± 2.18	20.74 ± 2.31
At registration:			
Gestation (d)	126.2 ± 41.9	122.6 ± 43.6	118.1 ± 43.6
Weight (lb)	120.9 ± 14.7	120.0 ± 14.0	120.0 ± 14.2
Arm girth (cm)	23.9 ± 2.6	23.7 ± 2.4	24.0 ± 2.6
Triceps skinfold (mm)	14.4 ± 6.0	14.2 ± 5.9	14.5 ± 6.3
Subscapular skinfold (mm)	12.4 ± 4.7	12.1 ± 4.8	12.2 ± 5.1
# cigarettes/d	4.6 ± 8.0	4.2 ± 7.4	3.7 ± 6.7
≥15 cigarettes/d (%)	10.4%	12.1%	7.2%
Calories, prior 24 hr	1,794 ± 775	1,912* ± 877	1,696* ± 866
Protein, prior 24 hr (gm)	66.4 ± 34.3	69.1 ± 37.5	60.7 ± 37.1
Low protein criterion (%)	47.4	45.3	50.4
Low weight gain criterion (%)	73.5	73.8	73.5
n	249	256	264

Means ± SD, except when indicated as (%), for 769 liveborn singletons (one woman who bore infant with Down syndrome omitted), by treatment group.
[a]For multiparae only; [b]among native born; *differences from rest of study population, p < 0.05.

significantly lower in the Complement group, but neither mean height nor reported weight at conception was significantly different among the three groups. The women in the Control group, when compared to those in the two other groups combined, reported having taken significantly fewer calories and less protein during the 24 hours prior to recruitment. The women in the Complement group reported having taken significantly more calories. Since initial dietary intake, independent of other characteristics, was not related to birthweight, these differences are of doubtful importance. The characteristics that might be expected to relate to perinatal outcome (history of past low birthweight, maternal weight, weight gain to the time of recruitment) did not differ significantly among the treatment groups.

CONCLUSION

From the above data we conclude that the design of this study was accomplished. The numbers of women recruited yielded a number of liveborn singletons closely in accord with requirements of the values set for hypothesis-testing. Losses among the women recruited did not produce detectable biases of concern to the analysis. In particular, voluntary discontinuation of beverage did not affect either of the two groups assigned to beverages disproportionately. These matters are crucial to the design and execution of experimental studies. The material presented in this chapter allows us to assert that in terms of the prerequisites of hypothesis-testing and unbiased sampling the study described is a valid experiment.

SUMMARY

The design of a randomized controlled trial of nutritional supplementation in pregnancy is described. The object of the trial was to accelerate fetal growth, raise birthweight, and influence the development of the offspring. The magnitude of the effect on birthweight aimed for was 125 gm. A test of an effect of this size with an alpha level of 0.05 and a power of

0.80 required a sample size of approximately 750. A total of 1,051 women were recruited into the study; 814 stayed active to delivery; 770 delivered liveborn singletons.

The 814 women active at delivery were distributed across treatment groups as follows: 263 to the high protein Supplement; 272 to the balanced Complement that provided much less protein and somewhat fewer calories; 279 to the nonintervention Control group. The experimental population at delivery was depleted by 121 women who, after agreeing to participate, were subsequently not activated into the study; 14 who were discontinued for medical reasons; 43 who moved from the New York area; 59 who discontinued the regiment of supplements; and 36 fetal deaths. Nine women bore twins.

Chapter II

The Monitoring of Experimental Intervention

MONITORING

The most elegant design of a study does not ensure its adequate execution. In many studies, experimental as well as observational, the fact that the intended treatment or exposure took place rests on questionable assumptions. Researchers as well as clinicians, as they moved out of hospital wards to work among ambulatory subjects, have been chastened by a growing literature on noncompliance with treatment.

In few fields is the measurement of exposure to the factor under study more difficult than with the nutritional intake of free-living populations. The 24-hour dietary recall, the most useful available measure, has seldom been validated or tested for reliability. No one would claim that a single 24-hour period gives an adequate measure of the regular diet of given individuals. Longer periods are subject to severe problems of recall, while attempts to measure directly the food eaten are altogether too laborious for large field studies. Moreover, even when compliance with prescribed food supplements is under direct observation, there is often no assurance that the supplement did not merely replace other items in the regular diet. The result is that few studies of the effects of diet, under the conditions of daily life, have established their validity.

Therefore, when we undertook a trial of the effects of nutritional supplementation in pregnancy that was to require a large investment of research time and funds and, by the nature of things, was to last several years, we took pains to determine the level of supplementation achieved. The credibility of the study as a valid experiment depends on the demonstration that nutritional intervention took place as planned. To establish that the experimental exposure occurred, we devised several means of monitoring intake, and in addition used maternal weight gain as an index of adherence to supplementation.

Indices of Adherence to Treatment: Description

Beverage use was monitored in four ways. The first two were based on anamnestic indices. The other two were based on direct observation.

Quantitative 24-hour dietary recall. At registration in the study, 2 weeks later, again 4 weeks after that, and then close to the 32nd week of pregnancy, a quantitative 24-hour dietary recall was obtained by an experienced graduate nutritionist. She coded type and amounts of food eaten. Her coding was checked independently by a second nutritionist. We used the standardized format of the Ten State Nutrition Survey (U.S. DHEW, 1972), with which the senior nutritionist had long experience. The recalls gave estimates of the intake of 17 nutrients; they were analyzed by computer, from food composition tables adapted to the dietary customs of this population from those of the Ten State Survey. Adequate data were available for 714 of the 769 women who had liveborn singletons. We shall present here only the data for calories and protein, using the mean of all dietary recalls taken after registration.

Direct structured questioning. At every return clinic visit, scheduled at least once a month, each participant assigned to a dietary supplement was questioned about her ingestion of beverages over the preceding 24 hours, over the preceding week, and over the 3 weeks preceding that week. She was also asked about any problems encountered with their use. This history was taken by a trained health aide, who did not have access to the 24-hour dietary recall. We present here the data for intake on the previous day and the previous week, using mean values of all reports.

Inventory of unused beverage (can count). At each monthly delivery of beverage, the cans remaining in the home of the participant were counted. This count gave us an indication of maximum possible use. Inventory-taking was begun partway through the study.

Urinary riboflavin assay. Each can of beverage contained 7.5 mg of riboflavin.* This level is within the therapeutic dose, and was considered by our nutritional and obstetric consultants and reviewers to be entirely innocuous. At each clinic visit, scheduled at least once a month, urine specimens were requested from participants receiving beverage. These specimens were analyzed for riboflavin concentration. For any given woman in this analysis, we used the logarithm of the mean of all urinary riboflavin measurements.

Indices of Adherence to Treatment: Interrelationships

The four measures of adherence to treatment are complementary and supportive of each other, but each is a distinctive measure based on different kinds of evidence obtained by different observers, and the data they yield refer to different time periods of food and supplement consumption. Thus each index of adherence stands as a measure of a different if overlapping slice of behavior or metabolic process. Only the two anamnestic indices of beverage use in the previous 24 hours, obtained by the nutritionist and health aide respectively, offer alternative techniques for measuring the same issue. Even these do not all refer to the same days.

In the analysis of the anamnestic data on intake, for instance, we depend on a summation of diet recalls. These histories, which were taken at fairly long intervals but covered short periods (most often 24 hours) of the time intervening between recalls, perforce described continuous functions (average use throughout the period of participation in the study). Since these summations derive neither from the same forms of data collection nor from the identical time periods as other indices of diet intake, correlations among them can only indicate a

---

*The additional riboflavin was inadvertently omitted by the manufacturers from one batch of Complement used over a period of about six months. We were unable, in retrospect, to identify the women who received the batch which lacked riboflavin. This omission could only have weakened the observed (significant) relationships between urinary riboflavin and both the anamnestic measures.

degree of consistency of maternal beverage intake, and will support the validity of the measures more than they do their reliability.*

Again, in the analysis of observed data on intake, the urinary riboflavin level is not an equivalent expression of any other index of adherence. Insofar as riboflavin levels correlate with the other variables, these correlations also estimate validity of the anamnestic indices, and not reliability. The other observed index, the inventory of unused cans taken at each home delivery, is a measure of maximum possible use averaged over the entire period of study. Here again the correlations between the can count and the anamnestic indices can be taken as a validation of the anamnestic indices.

DIET INTAKE

Intercorrelations of Beverage Intake Indices

The correlation matrix of indices of beverage intake (Table 2.1) shows strong associations among the anamnestic indices and also, if somewhat less strong, among anamnestic and observed indices. This pattern accords with what might be expected given the nature of the measures. The intercorrelations between the anamnestic measures of beverage intake taken by the nutritionist and by the health aides are all higher than $r = 0.5$ ($p < 0.001$). These correlations do give some estimate of reliability. Exact replication is not to be expected since, as noted, some of the histories taken by the two different observers do not refer to the same day. The correlations are compatible with reasonable interobserver reliability as well as with consistency over time in the reported intake of each participant.

---

*An index is *valid*, in the simplest sense, to the degree that it does indeed measure the property that it purports to measure; validity must be tested against some criterion external to the index, for instance consensus of experts, coherence with other phenomena, confirmation by subsequent outcome, or another criterion "more valid" than the index. An index is *reliable* to the degree that in the measurement of a given property the result is reproducible; reliability is tested against repeated measurements, for instance on more than one occasion, or by more than one observer, or with more than one instrument.

TABLE 2.1. Indices of Beverage Intake

	Can count	Log mean urine riboflavin	Average no. cans/day: Health aide's history		Average no. cans/day: Health aide's history
			Previous 24 hr		Previous week
Log mean urine riboflavin	0.06 (263)	—	—		—
Average no. cans/day: Health aide's history					
previous 24 hr	0.21^c (287)	0.17^c (406)			—
previous work	0.13^a (286)	0.15^b (406)	0.81^c (435)		—
Average calories from beverage: Nutritionist's 24-hr diet recall	0.12^a (301)	0.16^b (391)	0.56^c (419)		0.56^c (418)

$^a p < 0.05.$
$^b p < 0.01.$
$^c p < 0.001.$

Intercorrelations of five indices of beverage intake among all women in the two treatment groups assigned to beverage (numbers for each correlation in parentheses).

The correlations between the anamnestic and observed indices of compliance with beverage regimen are satisfactory when taken as a whole. Thus, among all supplemented women (that is, taking the values of the row totals, in the column for the two beverage groups combined in Table 2.2) all six of the associations between anamnestic and observed indices were statistically significant. When the two beverage groups are separated, however, the correlations of urine riboflavin with anamnestic indices are seen to be quite different. The significant association is seen to reside entirely in the Complement group (Table 2.2). In the Supplement group correlations of urinary riboflavin were not significant for any of the three anamnestic indices.

By contrast, correlations of the anamnestic indices with can count, the other observed index, were not higher for the Complement than for the Supplement group. We infer that the lack of correlation of the anamnestic indices with urine riboflavin in the Supplement group does not invalidate those histories, but rather that the marker did not function as expected in the Supplement group. *Actual* urinary riboflavin levels in the Supplement group were high. That is, the singular lack of association in the Supplement group between histories of beverage intake and riboflavin levels in the urine is not a mere reflection of either noncompliance or measurement error. More likely, above a threshold value of riboflavin ingestion, metabolic factors override intake in determining excretion rates.

In this regard, the patterns of results among cohorts classified by stage of gestation at entry to treatment (entry cohort) are informative (Table 2.2). Among the two Supplement cohorts entering earliest (<15 weeks) and latest (25+ weeks), the correlation between urinary riboflavin and reports of beverage intake were near zero or negative. Yet mean values of urinary riboflavin were distinctly high among these two cohorts (3,006 mcg/ml and 3,299 mcg/ml, respectively). Among the two cohorts entering midway (between 15 and 24 weeks), on the other hand, the correlations of urinary riboflavin with histories of Supplement intake were satisfactory (r = 0.33 and 0.21 respectively for nutritionist's recall). Yet mean values of urinary riboflavin were much lower among these cohorts (1,858 mcg/ml

TABLE 2.2. Validation of Anamnestic Indices of Compliance With Treatment

		Reports of beverage intake											
		a) Nutritionists' diet recall: Average calories from beverage						b) Health aides' questionnaire of compliance: Average daily beverage intake					
		Preceding 24 hours			Preceding week			Preceding 24 hours			Preceding week		
Observed Indices	Entry cohort (gestation in weeks)	Supplement	Complement	Combined	Supplement	Complement	Combined	Supplement	Complement	Combined	Supplement	Complement	Combined
Can count	<15	0.25	0.15	0.16	0.36[b]	0.15	0.16	0.18	0.27[b]	0.27[a]	0.03	0.17
	15–	0.02	0.23	0.11	0.10			0.25	0.17	−0.16	0.30	0.18
	20–	0.19	0.06	0.09	0.19			0.11	0.15	0.11	0.03	0.07
	25+	−0.08	0.11	0.04	0.14			0.22	0.12	0.25	0.04	0.10
	Total	0.12	0.14	0.12[a]	0.22[b]			0.19[a]	0.21[c]	0.15	0.11	0.13[a]
Urine riboflavin	<15	−0.13	0.23[a]	0.07	−0.02			0.29[b]	0.13	0.06	0.21	0.12
	15–	0.33[a]	0.14	0.21[a]	0.17			0.22	0.20[a]	0.17	0.17	0.16
	20–	0.21	0.26	0.26[a]	0.16			0.16	0.16	0.24	0.08	0.15
	25+	−0.09	0.36	0.18	−0.02			0.62[b]	0.15	−0.09	0.63[b]	0.22
	Total	0.08	0.22[b]	0.16[b]	0.08			0.26[c]	0.17[c]	0.09	0.20[b]	0.15[a]

[a] $p < 0.05$.
[b] $p < 0.01$.
[c] $p < 0.001$.

Correlations, within treatment groups and entry cohorts, between reports of beverage intake (nutritionists' diet recall and health aide's questionnaire) and observed indices of intake (count of unused cans, and log mean urine riboflavin) for mothers of liveborn singletons.

and 1,866 mcg/ml) than among the early and late entering cohorts. Out-of-range riboflavin values were not responsible for undermining the anamnestic/riboflavin correlations; standard deviations of the riboflavin values were much the same in the four entry cohorts.

That metabolic processes over and above intake influence riboflavin excretion may also be inferred from the contrasting riboflavin/anamnestic correlations of the Supplement and Complement groups. In the Supplement group correlations are strongest among the midgestation entry cohorts; in the Complement group by far the strongest correlations occur among the early and late entry cohorts.

The pattern of correlations of anamnestic indices with can count is markedly different from that with riboflavin. While the overall correlations noted above are all satisfactory, the size of the correlations declines fairly consistently with successively later entry to treatment. This result can be attributed to increasing insensitivity of can count as a measure with enrollment late in pregnancy; the later the enrollments the fewer home deliveries of cans and the fewer counts are made. Nutritionists and health aide histories were less affected, since clinic visits are stepped up late in pregnancy.

Estimates of Beverage Intake, and Substitution of Regular Diet

The estimates of beverage intake were similar for each of the three data sources from which they derived (Table 2.3). Data from each source were converted into an estimate of average daily caloric and protein intake. In the light of the differences in these data sources described above, the similarity of estimated intake is notable. The range of estimated average intake for all three sources is 69% to 79% of the prescribed amount for Supplement (326 to 370 of the 470 calories) and 69% to 79% for Complement (233 to 254 of the 322 calories).

The Supplement group, on average, reported taking 326 calories a day from beverage, according to the nutritionists' 24 hour diet recalls: 261 (or 80%) of these calories were over and above the reported intake of the Control group. Thus 65 calories (or 20%) could be considered as substituting for cal-

TABLE 2.3. Diet Intake During Study by Treatment Group

	Supplement		Complement		Controls	
	Calories	Protein (gm)	Calories	Protein (gm)	Calories	Protein (gm)
1) Nutritionists' 24-hr diet recalls:						
Beverage alone	326 ± 157	28 ± 13	233 ± 118	5 ± 3		
Exclusive of beverage	2,000 ± 739	74 ± 28	2,039 ± 765	79 ± 31		
Total	2,326 ± 764	102 ± 32	2,272 ± 773	83 ± 31	2,065 ± 699	79 ± 29
2) Health aides' questionnaires of beverage used:						
Preceding 24 hr	370 ± 170	31 ± 14	254 ± 116	5 ± 2		
Preceding week	346 ± 132	29 ± 11	234 ± 92	4 ± 2		
3) Count of residual cans	359 ± 122	31 ± 10	244 ± 85	5 ± 2		

Average daily caloric and protein intake of mothers of liveborn singletons during study estimated from 1) nutritionists' 24-hour diet recalls for beverage alone (n = 455), intake other than beverage, and total intake (n = 714), 2) health aides' history of beverage intake in preceding 24 hours (n = 465) and preceding week; and 3) residual can count (n = 323).

ories that would otherwise have been taken in the regular diet. The Complement group reported taking 233 calories a day from beverage. Two hundred and seven (or 89%) of these calories were over and above the reported intake of the Control group, and 26 calories (or 11%) could be considered as substituting for the regular diet. The mean caloric intake of Controls (2,065 calories/day) was low when compared with the 1968 United States National Academy of Sciences National Research Council Recommended Daily Allowance (RDA) in pregnancy, which is about 2,400 calories a day.

The reported mean intake of protein in the Supplement group was 101.9 gm/day, a value in the range reported among the most affluent populations. The Supplement group thus achieved the intended level for the study. The intake of protein exclusive of beverage was 74.2 gm/day. The reported mean protein intake in the Complement group was 82.7 gm/day, of which 78.2 gm were exclusive of beverage. The reported mean protein intake among Controls was 79.3 gm/day, a level distinctly higher than might have been expected in this economically marginal population. The reported levels in the study are not consistent with our starting assumption that the target population was deprived of protein. The 1968 Recommended Daily Allowance, current at the outset of the study, was 65 gm/day, and the 1974 RDA is 76 gm. Thus, the calorie intake of the target population was low, but the protein intake was not.

The measure of diet intake, an average of all recalls, can be expected to vary by the stage of gestation at which a woman enters the study. For early-entering cohorts, the measure covers a greater part of pregnancy than for late-entering cohorts. In general, the earlier in pregnancy that treatment began, the greater the difference in reported caloric and protein intake between the two treatment groups and the Control group (Tables 2.4 and 2.5, Fig. 2.1). The narrowing of differences with progressively later registration among the two late-entry cohorts of the beverage treatment groups and Controls was the consequence of a decline in the treated groups in the intake of food other than that of the nutritional supplements. Thus, if the calories provided by the beverages are excluded, in the Supplement group the cohort registered between 25–29 weeks

TABLE 2.4. Caloric Intake

Gestation at registration (weeks)	Treatment group			Total
	Supplement	Complement	Controls	
1) Total with beverage				
<15	2,254 ± 739 (77)	2,260 ± 805 (90)	2,025 ± 677 (108)	2,166 ± 747 (275)
15–19	2,498 ± 786 (60)	2,344 ± 799 (58)	2,090 ± 576 (66)	2,303 ± 742 (184)
20–24	2,254 ± 740 (53)	2,311 ± 781 (54)	2,105 ± 751 (44)	2,231 ± 763 (151)
25+	2,276 ± 772 (37)	2,120 ± 579 (31)	2,123 ± 925 (29)	2,179 ± 768 (97)
Total	2,326 ± 764 (231)	2,272 ± 773 (234)	2,065 ± 699 (249)	2,217 ± 754 (714)
2) Without beverage				
<15	1,952 ± 706	2,037 ± 795	2,025	2,009 ± 726
15–19	2,152 ± 761	2,101 ± 783	2,090	2,114 ± 708
20–24	1,905 ± 744	2,069 ± 737	2,105	2,022 ± 749
25+	1,969 ± 728	1,890 ± 629	2,123	1,990 ± 764
Total	2,000 ± 739	2,039 ± 760	2,065	2,035 ± 733
3) Beverage alone				
<15	301 ± 147	223 ± 104	0	
15–19	345 ± 165	242 ± 111	0	
20–24	349 ± 135	242 ± 142	0	
25+	307 ± 184	230 ± 124	0	
Total	326 ± 157	233 ± 118	0	

Reported daily calorie intake (± SD) while in study estimated from nutritionists' diet history: 1) total with beverage; 2) without beverage; and 3) beverage alone, by treatment group and entry cohort, among mothers of liveborn singletons (8 cases deviant for birthweight by gestation included only in Total rows). Numbers of women in parentheses.

TABLE 2.5. Protein Intake

Gestation at registration (weeks)	Treatment group			
	Supplement	Complement	Controls	Total
1) Total with beverage				
<15	97.6 ± 42.0 (76)	83.1 ± 32.1 (90)	80.3 ± 30.9 (108)	86.0 ± 32.3 (274)
15–19	108.9 ± 33.2 (59)	84.3 ± 29.1 (58)	79.1 ± 27.1 (66)	90.4 ± 32.5 (182)
20–24	100.6 ± 29.4 (53)	84.9 ± 34.3 (54)	77.5 ± 26.4 (44)	88.3 ± 31.9 (151)
25+	100.2 ± 35.0 (37)	74.9 ± 25.2 (31)	79.1 ± 32.3 (29)	85.9 ± 31.3 (97)
Total	101.9 ± 32.4 (229)	82.7 ± 31.2 (234)	79.3 ± 29.3 (248)	87.7 ± 32.5 (711)
2) Without beverage				
<15	72.2 ± 16.7	78.9 ± 32.1	80.3	77.6 ± 30.4
15–19	79.2 ± 28.3	79.5 ± 28.5	79.1	79.3 ± 27.9
20–24	71.0 ± 27.7	80.2 ± 33.6	77.5	76.2 ± 29.9
25+	74.0 ± 29.4	70.6 ± 25.9	79.1	74.5 ± 29.3
Total	74.2 ± 28.0	78.2 ± 30.9	79.3	77.3 ± 29.5
3) Beverage alone				
<15	25.6 ± 12.5	4.2 ± 2.0		
15–19	29.3 ± 14.1	4.8 ± 2.9		
20–24	29.7 ± 11.5	4.7 ± 3.1		
25+	26.2 ± 15.6	4.3 ± 2.3		
Total	27.7 ± 13.3	4.5 ± 2.6		

Reported daily protein intake (gm ± SD) while in study estimated from nutritionists' diet recalls: 1) total with beverage; 2) without beverage; and 3) beverage alone, by treatment group and entry cohort, among mothers of liveborn singletons (8 cases deviant for birthweight by gestation included only in Total rows). Numbers of women in parentheses.

Monitoring of Experimental Intervention / 39

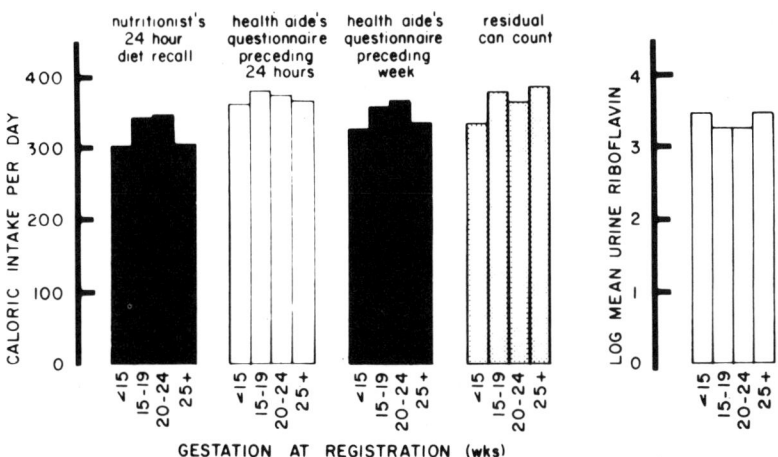

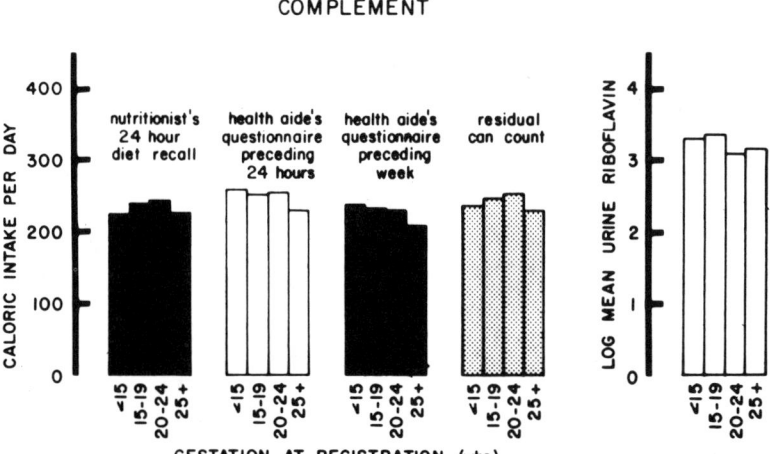

Fig. 2.1. Estimates of intake supplied by beverages, among entry cohorts, according to several indices. a) Supplement; b) Complement.

gestation reported taking an average of 154 fewer calories in their regular daily diet than did Controls. In the Complement group, this cohort took 234 fewer calories than the Controls. Despite the narrowing of the gap between treatment groups and Controls in the late entry cohorts, the reported use of supplementation was maintained with consistency in all entry cohorts (Tables 2.4–2.6; Figs. 2.1 and 2.2).

A few characteristics of the women were related to beverage intake (Table 2.7). In both treatment groups, age was significantly related to three of the five indices of intake studied. Duration of education was significantly related to urine riboflavin levels, although not to the remaining four indices. Heavy smoking was negatively correlated with nutritionist's history of Supplement intake. The few significant correlations with reported beverage use tended to be of low magnitude and without recognizable pattern. Age, education, and these other characteristics were distributed evenly among the treatment groups. Thus, the differences in the use of the two beverages among participants do not affect the inferences to be drawn from the nutritional experiment.

For the same reason, the association of prior characteristics with reported total dietary intake of calories and protein should not affect inference. Among Controls alone, total dietary in-

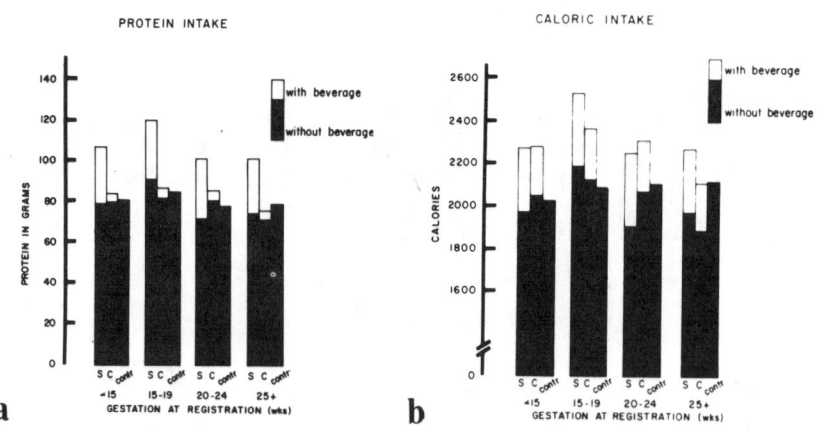

Fig. 2.2. Estimates of total daily diet intake among entry cohorts for each treatment group. a) Protein; b) Caloric intake.

take was significantly associated with age, with marriage, with being a student, and with occupational status. These associations were not found in the two supplemented groups. Nutritional supplements seem to have overridden the influence of such factors on dietary intake.

WEIGHT GAIN

Indices of Weight Gain

Maternal weight gain is a potential mediator of fetal growth. It is also the most reliably measured criterion of effective dietary intervention. Three variables are used in the following analysis to represent maternal weight gain during pregnancy.

1) Total Weight Gain is defined as the difference between the weight recorded at last clinic visit and the reported weight at conception. Total Weight Gain therefore includes some weight gained before recruitment into the study, as well as weight gained during the study.

2) Average Weight Gain is defined as the average number of pounds per week gained during enrollment in the study. This variable reflects weight gain during participation in the study only. The variable was derived by subtracting the weight recorded at the registration visit from that at last clinic visit, and dividing by the time interval between the two visits.

3) Early Weight Gain is defined as the average pounds per week gained during the first month after registration in the study. The variable was derived by subtracting the weight recorded at registration from the clinic weight taken closest in time to a point four weeks after registration (range 3–7 weeks), and dividing by the time interval between the two observations. This variable is meant to reflect the response of weight gain to the initiation of treatment.

Early Weight Gain and Average Weight Gain, unlike Total Weight Gain, are affected by stage of gestation at entry into the study, since the rate of weight gain increases after the first trimester. On the other hand, and again unlike Total Weight Gain, Early Weight Gain and Average Weight Gain are not only exclusive of weight gain prior to recruitment in the study, but they are largely independent of duration of gestation at delivery.

TABLE 2.6. Beverage Intake by Stage of Gestation at Entry to Study

Gestation at registration (weeks)	Mean calorie intake per day				Log mean urine riboflavin
	Nutritionists' 24-hour diet recall	Health aides' questionnaire		Residual can count	
		Preceding 24 hours	Preceding week		
Supplement					
<15	301 ± 147 (77)	362 ± 165 (76)	328 ± 129 (76)	335 ± 118 (59)	3.48 ± 0.53 (72)
15–19	345 ± 165 (60)	380 ± 144 (60)	359 ± 114 (60)	376 ± 123 (48)	3.27 ± 0.55 (56)
20–24	349 ± 135 (53)	376 ± 173 (47)	365 ± 126 (47)	363 ± 116 (38)	3.27 ± 0.60 (43)
25+	307 ± 184 (37)	366 ± 224 (29)	335 ± 168 (28)	384 ± 116 (27)	3.49 ± 0.46 (26)
Total	327 ± 157 (231)	370 ± 170 (215)	346 ± 132 (214)	359 ± 122 (173)	3.38 ± 0.55 (199)
Complement					
<15	223 ± 104 (90)	260 ± 108 (90)	239 ± 80 (90)	239 ± 79 (56)	3.31 ± 0.49 (85)
15–19	242 ± 111 (58)	252 ± 124 (57)	235 ± 90 (57)	248 ± 83 (31)	3.34 ± 0.54 (55)
20–24	242 ± 142 (54)	253 ± 133 (51)	232 ± 106 (51)	254 ± 74 (41)	3.12 ± 0.62 (47)
25+	230 ± 124 (31)	231 ± 143 (22)	211 ± 105 (22)	231 ± 111 (22)	3.17 ± 0.54 (20)
Total	233 ± 118 (234)	254 ± 121 (221)	234 ± 92 (221)	244 ± 85 (150)	3.26 ± 0.55 (208)

Four estimates of average daily calorie intake from beverage only, and log mean urine riboflavin (± SD) by treatment group and entry cohort among liveborn singletons (8 cases with birthweight deviant for gestation included only in Total rows). Numbers of women in parentheses.

TABLE 2.7. Beverage Use by Prior Maternal Characteristics

	Average daily calories from beverage, nutritionists' 24-hr diet recall			Average daily beverage use, health aides' questionnaire						Average daily beverage use, residual can count			Log mean urinary riboflavin		
				Prior 24 hours			Prior week								
	Supp	Comp	Total	Supp	Comp	Total	Supp	Comp	Total	Supp	Comp	Total	Supp	Comp	Total
Mother's age (yr)				0.07	0.17	0.12[a]	0.03	0.24[c]	0.14[b]				0.28[c]	0.09	0.17[c]
Parity (n)													0.17[a]	0.02	0.10
Primigravidae vs others													−0.14	−0.09	−0.10[a]
Past neonatal death[d] (n)													0.04	0.20[a]	0.11
Married vs others													0.12	0.13	0.12[a]
Foreign vs native born										0.10	0.19[a]	0.14[b]	0.17[a]	0.14[a]	0.15[b]
Education (yr)															
Occupational status maternal grandfather													−0.15	0.20[a]	0.03
Income per person													−0.09	−0.15[a]	−0.10[a]
Students vs others							−0.01	−0.14[a]	−0.08	−0.17[a]	−0.03	−0.10			
At conception:															
weight							0.03	0.14[a]	0.08	0.09	0.20[a]	0.14[b]			
ponderal index										0.08	0.19[a]	0.10			
At registration:															
gestation				0.14[a]	−0.02	0.06				0.20[b]	−0.01	0.09			
weight										0.07	0.15	0.11[a]			
arm girth										0.07	0.19[a]	0.13[a]			
calories, prior 24 hr				−0.11	−0.12	−0.10[a]				−0.19[a]	−0.09	−0.14[a]			
15+ cigarettes/day				0.09	0.12	0.10	0.02	0.13[a]	0.07						
low protein criterion	−0.14[a]	0.05	−0.06												
low weight gain criterion										−0.01	−0.21[a]	−0.10			

Use of nutritional supplements during study correlated with characteristics of subjects at or before recruitment into the study, by treatment group.
(Entries omitted if no significant correlates in row.)
[a] $p < 0.05$.
[b] $p < 0.01$.
[c] $p < 0.001$.
[d] Multigravidae only.

Treatment Effects on Weight Gain*

Total Weight Gain, Average Weight Gain, and Early Weight Gain each show a slight gradient between the treated and control groups, generally declining from Supplement, through Complement to Control. For Supplement, Complement, and Control respectively, Total Weight Gain is 23.3 pounds, 23.4 pounds, and 21.6 pounds; Average Weight Gain is 0.96, 0.95, and 0.91 pounds; and Early Weight Gain is 0.99, 0.89, and 0.85 pounds. Only Early Weight Gain, however, shows a significant treatment effect in favor of Supplement over Control ($t = 2.01$, $p < 0.05$).

In view of their influence on weight gain, and on birthweight as the central outcome measure, duration of gestation at entry to treatment and at delivery were introduced into the analysis, specified as "entry cohort" and as "prematurity/maturity" respectively. When the groups are categorized by entry cohort, significant treatment effects in the expected direction are found for each index, but they are all confined to the earliest entry cohort (<15 weeks gestation).

When the groups are categorized by prematurity/maturity, a striking divergence in Total Weight Gain and Average Weight Gain appears between women delivered at term and those delivered prematurely. The entire positive treatment effect noted in the early entry cohort is confined to women delivered at term (Appendix 2.1c). Among women delivered prematurely, the Supplement group is at a distinct disadvantage in Total Weight Gain and Average Weight Gain, although numbers are too small for the result to reach a level of statistic significance. It is notable that for Early Weight Gain, the gradient across treatment groups remains unaffected by duration of gestation at delivery (Appendix 2.1b).

These results give a strong indication that a disturbance of weight gain occurred among women treated with Supplement who delivered their infants prematurely, and who were exposed to Supplement treatment early in pregnancy. These women, like those who went to term, had high Early Weight Gain; later they lost their early advantage and gained less than the women in the other two treatment groups, and by the time of delivery they had markedly depressed weight gain.

*See Appendix 2.1.

Dietary Intake and Weight Gain (Table 2.8)

Coherence among indices of dietary intake and indices of weight gain could lend further validity to our assumptions about treatment effects. In pursuit of this aim, we consider mainly the correlations of Average Weight Gain with the average intake reported in the 24-hour dietary recalls, and the correlations of Early Weight Gain with the concurrent 24-hour dietary recall, that is, the first recall after initiation of treatment.

Average Weight Gain was significantly related to reported average daily intake of calories ($r = 0.11$, $p < 0.01$) and protein ($r = 0.11$, $p < 0.01$) and to average daily calories and protein derived exclusively from supplementary beverages (for both, $r = 0.10$, $p < 0.05$).* The Supplement group contributed virtually the entirety of these significant associations. The earliest entry cohort was mainly responsible, further evidence that weight gain was far more responsive to diet level in the first trimester of pregnancy than later. Early Weight Gain was significantly related to diet intake measured at the same time. The correlation with calories and protein reported at the first dietary recall taken after recruitment into the study was $r = 0.10$ ($p < 0.05$). This first postregistration recall was scheduled between two to four weeks after recruitment into the study. Early Weight Gain was significantly related also to log mean urinary riboflavin level ($r = 0.12$, $p < 0.05$), particularly among women on Supplement ($r = 0.18$, $p < 0.05$). The general pattern of the results confirms that both regular diet and diet supplementation accelerated weight gain, but that this effect was limited to those recruited in the first third of pregnancy.

We carried out several sets of multiple regression analyses in order to control potential confounding, and to detect suppressor and distorting factors in the treatment effects as well as interactions (Appendix 2.2). The factors chosen as independent variables were the stratifying conditions and other factors which

---

*Average Weight Gain was also significantly related to total calories and protein (for both, $r = 0.12$, $p < 0.01$) at the *first* postregistration dietary recall. The relation here was strongest among women receiving Complement (for calories, $r = 0.19$, $p < 0.01$; for protein, $r = 0.23$, $p < 0.001$). Thus, for the Complement group, diet intake in the period immediately after beginning treatment had a greater influence on weight gain averaged over the entire duration of the study than did the diet averaged over the same period. This sequence is consistent with a gradual alteration of metabolic pathways from diet intake to fetal growth in the Complement group (see below).

TABLE 2.8. Weight Gain and Dietary Intake

		Treatment groups			Duration of gestation at entry (weeks)			
	All women	Supplement	Complement	Control	<15	15–	20–	25–
a) Average Weight Gain (n = 741)								
Average diet recall, postregistration								
Calories	0.10[b]	0.13	0.08	0.07	0.16[b]	0.05	0.09	0.03
Protein	0.12[b]	0.17[b]	0.11	0.05	0.14[a]	0.19[a]	0.04	0.01
Beverage calories	0.09[a]	0.15[a]	0.02	–	0.06	0.15	0.00	0.14
Beverage protein	0.07	0.15[a]	0.02	–	0.03	0.21[a]	0.02	0.02
b) Early Weight Gain (n = 649)								
First diet recall postregistration								
Calories	0.10[a]	0.04	0.07	0.17[a]	0.12	–0.04	0.19[a]	–0.02
Protein	0.10[a]	0.04	0.14	0.09	0.14[a]	0.00	0.15	0.02
Beverage calories	0.05	0.07	0.02	–	0.09	0.05	0.00	–0.01
Beverage protein	0.08	0.07	0.05	–	0.12	0.13	–0.02	–0.07

a) Average Weight Gain and average intake; b) Early Weight Gain and early intake, correlated within treatment groups, and within cohorts defined by stage of gestation at recruitment, among woman delivering liveborn singletons.
[a] $p < 0.05$.
[b] $p < 0.01$.

related strongly to weight gain in pregnancy. These analyses do not require modification of the inferences drawn from the preceding tables:

1) Appendix 2.2a shows that the effect of Supplement on Early Weight Gain held, with many important and available potential confounding variables controlled.

2) Appendix 2.2b continues the analysis of Appendix 2.2a for four additional steps. These equations show that given a history of past low birthweight, Early Weight Gain was significantly greater for the Complement group than for Controls.

3) Appendix 2.2c shows that Average Weight Gain did not relate to treatment group after several characteristics present before treatment were controlled.

4) Appendix 2.2d continues the analysis in Appendix 2.2c for an additional 12 steps. An interaction occurs between treatment group and weight at conception: in the Complement group, the greater the weight of the woman at conception, the more was the Average Weight Gain.

5) Appendix 2.2e shows that reported caloric intake during the study, irrespective of treatment group, related significantly to Average Weight Gain. Protein intake did not account for Average Weight Gain over and above calorie intake.

DISCUSSION AND CONCLUSIONS

Nutritional Intake

Against the standard of the current National Academy of Sciences Recommended Daily Allowance for pregnant women, the reported dietary intake among Controls shows that the target population was calorie deprived and not protein deprived. This result contradicts prevalent beliefs as well as the preliminary data available to us for the target population at the time we began our survey.

All the available information indicates that the participants in this study cooperated with the prescribed treatment regimen to a satisfactory, indeed to a high, degree. Reported use of beverage by the participants can be taken as substantially accurate. Use was validated in several ways. Thus the data derived from the independent reports of intake gathered by the nutritionists and the health aides separately, and the two independently observed indices — excretion of excess riboflavin in the urine and inventory of unused cans — correlated with each other in a consistently significant and reasonably coherent manner. Allowances must be made, however, for some unusual fluctuations in riboflavin levels. These we think can best be attributed to variations in riboflavin metabolism both with stage of pregnancy and with the composition of nutritional supplements. That these two factors alter absorption, metabolism, or excretion is suggested by several additional kinds of data discussed later or still to be reported.

The measures of nutritional intake are all in good agreement about the amount of beverage actually taken. On average, about three-quarters of the prescribed amount of beverage was probably ingested. For the Supplement group we estimated, from the 24-hour dietary recalls, that 326 calories were derived daily from the beverage: 80% of these calories were over and above the expected regular diet and 20% were substituted for the regular diet. For the Complement group we estimated that 233 calories were derived daily from the beverage; 89% of these calories were over and above the expected regular diet, and 11% were substituted for the regular diet. The increment in total daily dietary intake among women receiving treatment compared with Controls was less marked among those registering for prenatal care later in pregnancy (after 19 weeks gestation) than among those registering earlier. The later registering supplemented women did not report a lower intake of beverage, but a lower intake of other food.

Gradients of diet intake found to be associated with sociodemographic factors in the Control group were not found in the two supplemented groups. These gradients were obliterated, we infer, by dietary treatment. In the Supplement group alone, however, and not in the Complement or Control groups, thinner and lighter women reported eating more than heavier and fatter women. The difference between the two supplemented groups in this regard is not readily explained.

Weight Gain

The indices of weight gain during pregnancy (Total Weight Gain, Average Weight Gain, Early Weight Gain) were consistently and significantly related to nutritional intervention. These indices of weight gain were also related to other indicators of dietary intake and supplementation, such as intake reported for the previous 24 hours, reported use of nutritional supplements, and excretion of riboflavin marker. The correlations of weight gain with these indicators were accounted for almost entirely by the high protein Supplement. It is far from apparent why the balanced supplementation provided by Complement should not, excepting in the period immediately after treatment began, have produced significant associations of diet intake measures with weight gain. The expected gradient of treatment effects on weight gain was found with the high protein Supplement showing the maximum effect, and the balanced Complement showing somewhat less of an effect.

Significant effects of treatment on weight gain, however, were limited to women recruited early in pregnancy, before 15 weeks gestation. Analysis by duration of gestation at delivery revealed a marked divergence in treatment effects on weight gain for two of the three weight gain indices. Early Weight Gain was high among women on Supplement recruited early in gestation, whatever the duration of gestation at delivery. Total and Average Weight Gain, too, were both high among early recruits on Supplement compared with those on Complement and Controls, but *only* if they had carried their infants to term. Women on Supplement who delivered prematurely (the evidence shows that very early delivery can best be construed as an untoward treatment effect) had lower Total and Average Weight Gains than women on Complement and Controls. Hence, the early recruits did not sustain their increments in weight gain.

Among those women on Supplement the data on weight gain (taken together with data on outcome still to be reported) point to a causal sequence in which the high protein Supplement, after inducing an initial acceleration in weight gain, then induced decelerated weight gain in a susceptible minority of women who delivered prematurely.

We take these results on weight gain as showing that the gradient in dietary intake aimed for and achieved across the three treatment groups was transmuted into gradients in maternal weight gain. This happened in complicated ways. Weight gain effects were conditional on stage of pregnancy at the outset of treatment, on duration of pregnancy, and on the composition of the beverage used. Like the indices of beverage use, the results support the conclusion that the nutritional experiment indeed took place. The data on diet intake and weight gain taken together show that the intention that the supplements be used in addition to regular diet was in general fulfilled. The intake of nutritional supplements can thus be held sufficient to afford a reasonable test of the initial hypotheses. Certainly specific subgroups, like the women recruited early in pregnancy who went to term, not only used the supplements as fully as one could hope, but responded as expected in terms of weight gain.

The limitations of the treatment effects on weight gain complicate interpretation of the experiment. We must cope with the weight gain response confined to women recruited early in pregnancy; with the absence of significant effects of the balanced Complement; and with the paradoxical results of the Supplement treatment among premature deliveries.

With regard to the stage of gestation at recruitment, women recruited late in pregnancy do not have unequivocal evidence of a level of supplementation adequate to test the initial hypotheses. Doubt arises among them on the single ground that the response of weight gain to treatment was poor. It does not follow that the *uptake* of treatment was poor, however. We considered three among several explanations for the disparate effects of treatment on weight gain between the cohorts recruited early in pregnancy and those recruited late.

1) Only the women recruited before 15 weeks gestation participated actively in the study and adhered to the regimen prescribed. The array of indices of dietary intake does not support this explanation, since there is no suggestion that reported intake of women recruited early in gestation was greater than that of women recruited late in gestation.

2) All those supplemented complied similarly with the regimen irrespective of gestation at recruitment, but the physiological response to the initiation of dietary supplementation was affected by the stage of gestation, and was diminished after the first trimester of pregnancy. In favor of this explanation we may note that among women recruited early in pregnancy, regular diet averaged throughout pregnancy related to Average Weight Gain. Among women recruited later in pregnancy, regular diet did not relate to weight gain. Collateral evidence also favors this explanation, in that it suggests that weight gain owed to fat deposition is complete by the middle or before the end of the second trimester, and that subsequent weight gain is owed to fluid retention and increases in the products of conception [Hytten and Leitch, 1971].

3) While both supplemented groups complied with the regimen, total diet intake of these two groups converged with that of the unsupplemented Controls among the later entry cohorts because the supplemented cohorts did not increase their regular food intake as did Controls. This third explanation is at first sight consistent with the trends of reported diet intake by stage of gestation at recruitment among the women assigned to beverage treatments. With later registration there was no trend towards increased food intake other than beverage as there was among Controls. The explanation can be at best a partial one, however. The relative reductions in food intake among late entry cohorts are small. Conversely, supplementation in the 15–19 week entry cohort resulted in large reported dietary increments without affecting weight gain.

With regard to the puzzling failure of the balanced supplementation of Complement to accelerate weight gain, we resort to a metabolic explanation. Since the experiment was double-blind in terms of beverages, there is every reason to accept as unbiased the estimates from the anamnestic and objective indices, all of which point to equally high intake of Complement and Supplement. Moreover, the Complement riboflavin marker shows stronger and much more consistent correlations with anamnestic data than does the Supplement marker. This result obtains despite the six-month period when the riboflavin marker was omitted from the Complement beverage. It cannot be attributed to deficient intake of Supplement, since absolute values of urinary riboflavin in the Supplement group were high. It is our conviction overall that the metabolic paths for the balanced Complement differed in some unknown way from those for the high protein Supplement.*

The experiments of Riopelle and colleagues with Rhesus monkeys provide some analogies with these results, and likewise warn against facile explanations [Riopelle, Hale, and Watts, 1976; Riopelle and Favrett, 1977]. They found, among monkeys receiving diets of 1, 2, or 4 gm protein/kg/day from the 30th day of pregnancy, that only those on 4 gm protein/kg/day had increased weight gain. Moreover, the monkeys on the high protein diet had shorter length of gestation at delivery (a result that is also congruent with ours). Our results for maternal weight gain seem even less aberrant when taken together with those of the Taiwan study initiated by the late Bacon Chow [Herriot, Hsueh, and Aitchison, 1978]. The mean maternal weight at term of women supplemented with 40 gm of protein and 800 calories daily was identical with that of controls supplemented with no protein and less than 40 calories daily. This occurred despite the exclusion from the analysis of women who took less than 50% of the supplement.

The *conditional* nature of the treatment effects on weight gain do not counter and scarcely detract from the evidence that effective intervention took place. This evidence rests first on multiple indices of supplement intake cross-validated among themselves. It rests second on weight gain responses to supplementation. Weight gain is an objective and reliable measure. As an index of nutritional intake, however, it is less direct than the indices of food intake. Before becoming manifest as maternal weight gain, the nutrients ingested must be absorbed and metabolized, balanced against energy expenditure, and distrib-

---

*In the chapter on outcomes at birth, and in later papers, we shall report further intriguing features specific to the Complement group. Outcomes within the Complement group differed from other groups in numerous ways, eg riboflavin correlation, placental biochemical responses to the diet, effects on length of gestation, in addition to the weight gain differences reported here. See, for instance, Appendix 6 on placental biochemistry.

uted among the growing fetus and the mother. It is hardly surprising that the correlates of weight gain with dietary intake are not simple and straightforward.

We conclude that adherence to the prescribed treatment regimens in this study was at the least satisfactory, and indeed excellent in the light of initial expectations. Few other studies, completed or in progress, have evidence of so large a supplementary diet intake, and only one other has been able to ensure objectivity of measures by the use of a double-blind control in a randomized experiment [Blackwell et al, 1973; Herriot, Hsueh and Aitchison, 1978]. In the light of effective dietary supplementation, we conclude further that this experiment can be seen to have posed a reasonable test of the questions it set out to answer, namely, whether prenatal nutritional supplementation in a poor urban population in the United States can promote fetal growth and postnatal development.

SUMMARY

In a randomized controlled trial of prenatal nutritional supplementation, an extensive effort was made to determine whether the degree of supplementation that took place was adequate to test the hypotheses of the study. Contrary to expectation, the target population appeared to be calorie and not protein deprived. Intake was monitored by 1) 24-hour dietary recalls taken by experienced nutritionists; 2) histories of the use of supplements taken by health aides; 3) inventories of unused cans of supplement taken at each home delivery; 4) levels of urinary riboflavin, riboflavin having been incorporated in the supplementary beverages as a marker. These measures were all in good agreement and cross-validation among them satisfactory. Average intake was estimated at 69% to 79% of the prescribed regimen for both supplements. For the high protein Supplement, an estimated 326 calories were taken daily from the beverage, 20% of which substituted for regular diet. For the balanced protein/calorie Complement, an estimated 233 calories were taken daily from the beverage, 11% of which substituted for regular diet.

Three indices of weight gain (Total, Average, Early) were significantly related to indices of dietary intake, but for two (Total and Average Weight Gain), only among women recruited before 15 weeks gestation. Among them the expected gradient in weight gain across treatment groups was found, with the high protein Supplement having the maximum effect, and indeed responsible for virtually all significant effects. No ready explanation is available for the lack of significant associations of weight gain with Complement, aside from the smaller amount of calories it supplied. Of three possible explanations, for the different responses of the two treatment groups, and particularly of early and late entry cohorts within the treatment groups 1) it is considered unlikely taht the later recruits failed to adhere to the treatment regimen; 2) it is considered likely that the stage of gestation at the initiation of supplementation determines the physiological responses to supplements; and 3) it can be at best a partial explanation that among later recruits supplements replace regular diet to a greater degree than among early recruits. Among premature deliveries the high protein Supplement was associated with high Early Weight Gain and depressed Average and Total Weight Gains. It seems likely that the Supplement, after accelerating weight gain at the outset among women recruited early in pregnancy, later in pregnancy inhibited weight gain among a group that then delivered prematurely.

The evidence indicates that adherence to the treatment regimen among the experimental population sufficed for a reasonable test of the initial hypothesis, that is, whether prenatal nutritional supplementation in a poor urban population in the United States can affect birthweight and subsequent development.

Chapter III

Outcome at Birth: Effects on Duration of Gestation, Mortality, and Size

We turn now to analyze the outcome at birth of this randomized controlled trial of prenatal nutritional supplementation. The outcomes reported are confined to three important areas, namely duration of gestation, perinatal mortality, and infant size at birth. Infant size is of course a function of both duration of gestation and fetal growth rate. Other outcomes, such as neurological state and maturity, neonatal state and behavior, and the weight, biochemical attributes, histomorphometry, and pathology of the placenta, will be described in later reports. Some data on findings in the placenta are included in Appendices 6, 7, and 8.

RESULTS

Duration of Gestation

Life table analysis is an accurate way of assessing variation among groups in length of gestation. The method takes account of losses and recruitments to the study populations at each stage of pregnancy. Figure 3.1 is drawn from life tables. The figure shows rates of delivery for all participants up to 37 weeks gestation, including dropouts up to the time they left the study, at given stages of gestation among the three treatment groups. The life tables have been statistically tested for differences by the method of Mantel and Haenszel [1959].

Differences between the life table curves are not statistically significant at any stage of gestation, although close to it (Appendix 3.1). The favorable χ^2 value of 3.60 for the comparison of the Complement group with the other two groups combined up to 37 weeks gestation is just short of the 5% level of statistical significance. Likewise, the accelerated

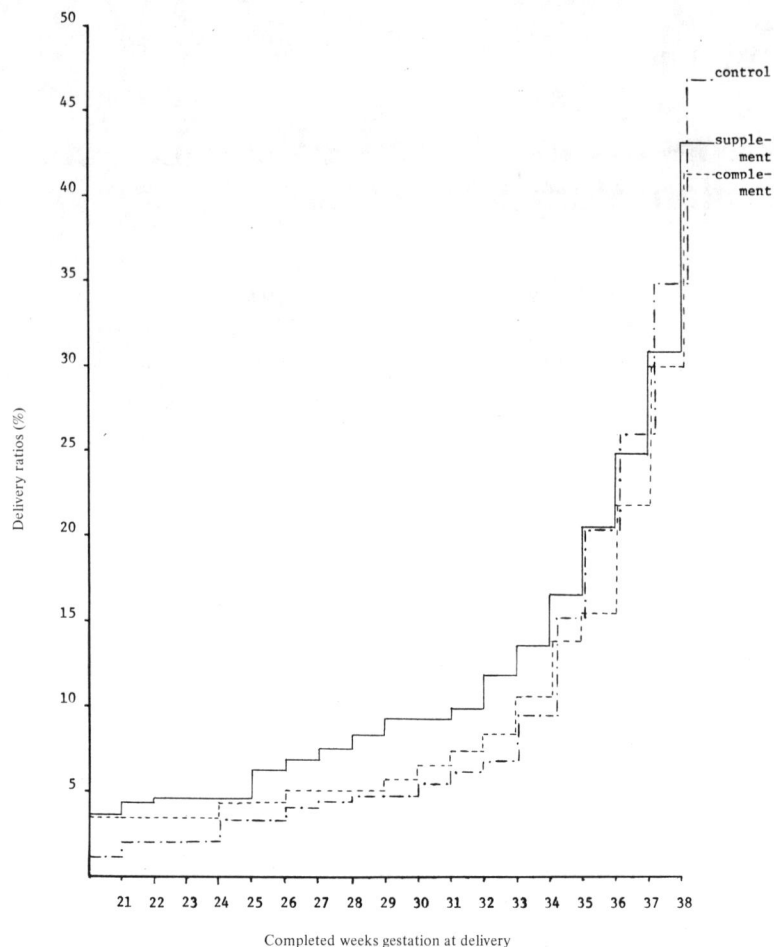

Fig. 3.1. Treatment and Prematurity. Cumulative rates of delivery (%) from life tables for each treatment group (see Appendix 3.1).

delivery rate between 25 and 30 weeks gestation in the Supplement group yields a χ^2 value of 3.51 (tested at the completion of 30 weeks gestation) for the comparison of the Supplement group with the other two groups combined. We shall see the importance of this result, even though short of statistical significance, when we turn to analyze neonatal deaths.

Dietary intake and extreme prematurity (Table 3.1). The 13 women in the Supplement group who delivered before 33 weeks gestation and for whom diet recalls were available reported taking more beverage (389 calories daily) than other women in that treatment group who delivered later (321 calories daily). At the same time they reported taking, on average, significantly fewer total calories each day than the other women in the same treatment group (1,912 vs 2,347, $t=2.01$, $p<0.05$) and markedly fewer calories over and above calories supplied by the beverage (1,523 vs 2,026 calories, $t=2.41$, $p<0.025$). The differences in protein intake varied in parallel with calories.

Very premature births in the Supplement group (≤ 33 weeks gestation at delivery), when compared with other premature births, were not uniquely associated either with high protein in the maternal diet or with low caloric intake (Table 3.2). What does distinguish the Supplement group of very early deliveries from the other groups is the *combination* of high protein with low caloric intake. Thus, these very premature deliveries occurred among a group of women who reduced their intake from regular diet. In the previous chapter, we noted that women on Supplement who delivered prematurely, after an initial spurt of weight gain similar to that of others on Supplement, later experienced a deceleration in weight gain.

Duration of gestation and maternal characteristics (Table 3.3). The relations of duration of gestation with maternal characteristics are somewhat diverse across treatment groups. In view of the excess of extreme prematurity in the Supplement group, it is of concern to discover whether in that group shortened gestation was associated with any special maternal attributes.

The following associations of duration of gestation were statistically significant *only* in the Supplement group:

1) with years of maternal education, $r = 0.15$ ($p < 0.05$);
2) with maternal ponderal index at conception, $r = 0.16$ ($p < 0.05$);
3) with being on welfare, $r = -0.15$ ($p < 0.05$);
4) among multiparae, with number of past low birthweight babies, $r = 0.29$ ($p < 0.01$).

By far the strongest correlation with prematurity in any treatment group is that of history of past low birthweight, which is significant only among women on Supplement.

Perinatal Mortality

Fetal deaths were defined to include all intrauterine deaths occurring at any stage of gestation (excluding only two ectopic pregnancies). Early fetal deaths were defined as those occurring up to and including 20 completed weeks of gestation from the date of last menstrual period. Late fetal deaths were defined as those occurring after 20 weeks of gestation. Neonatal deaths were defined as deaths in infants who showed any signs of life at birth, and who died by 28 days of age. In fact, there were no neonatal deaths after 8 days of life. Perinatal deaths were defined as the sum of late fetal deaths and neonatal deaths.

Table 3.4 gives crude fetal and neonatal death rates among those who were active to delivery. Table 3.4a includes twins, and Table 3.4b excludes them. Crude fetal death rates are almost identical among the 3 treatment groups, although slightly lower in the Supplement group (4.1%, 4.7%, and 4.3% in the Supplement, Complement, and Control groups respectively; excluding twins, 3.9%, 4.8% and 4.3% respectively).

The crude neonatal death rate was highest in the Supplement group. The difference between the crude neonatal death rate in the Supplement group and that of others hovered around the 5% level of statistical significance. For example, including twins, the Supplement group neonatal death rate was significantly higher than the Control group rate. Excluding twins, the neonatal death rate in the Supplement group was significantly high only in comparison with the other two groups combined.

To represent fully the experience of neonatal mortality in the study, life table analysis is necessary. Life tables can refer deaths that occur as gestation progresses to the population actually at risk, including women who did not complete the study regimen (Appendix 3.2 and Fig. 3.2). All the neonatal deaths occurred in infants delivered between 20 and 35 weeks gestation. Indeed all but three, one in each treatment group, occurred before 29 weeks gestation. Between 25 and 29 weeks

TABLE 3.1. Dietary and Beverage Intake and Prematurity

	A. Calories		B. Protein	
Treatment group	Early prematures	All others	Early prematures	All others
1. Intake including beverage:				
Supplement	(13) 1,912* ± 423	(214) 2,026** ± 773	91 ± 21	102 ± 33
Complement	(5) 2,772 ± 1,575	(228) 2,263 ± 743	96 ± 58	82 ± 30
Control	(6) 1,705 ± 743	(241) 2,077 ± 698	64 ± 26	81 ± 36
All	(24) 2,039 ± 949	(683) 2,224 ± 746	85 ± 36	88 ± 32
2. Intake excluding beverage:				
Supplement	1,523** ± 449	2,026** ± 744	58* ± 20	75* ± 28
Complement	2,531 ± 1,651	2,030 ± 726	91 ± 60	78 ± 30
Control	1,705 ± 743	2,077 ± 698	64 ± 26	81 ± 36
All	1,778 ± 985	2,045 ± 722	66 ± 36	78 ± 29
3. Beverage Intake				
Supplement	389 ± 82	321 ± 160	33 ± 7	27 ± 14
Complement	242 ± 125	233 ± 118	5 ± 2	4 ± 3

Average daily calories and grams of protein (calculated from nutritionist's 24 hour diet recalls) among early premature deliveries (≤ 32 weeks) and all others (≥ 33 weeks) by treatment groups, for all liveborn singletons with relevant data available except 8 deviant for length of gestation by birthweight. Numbers within parentheses equal number of women; ± = SD.

≤ 32 weeks vs ≥ 33 weeks for Supplement, *p < 0.05; **p < 0.025.

TABLE 3.2. Prematurity and Relative Protein Levels

	Supplement		Complement		Controls	
	Early prematures	Others	Early prematures	Others	Early prematures	Others
Total calories	1,912	2,347	2,772	2,263	1,705	2,077
% protein[a]	19.0	17.5	13.8	14.6	14.9	15.4
Ratio of % protein compared to controls delivered at 33+ weeks	1.22	1.14	0.90	0.95	0.97	1.0
Number	13	214	5	228	6	241

Percent calories of average total diet supplied by protein among early premature deliveries ($\leq$ 32 weeks) and others in three treatment groups, for all liveborn singletons with relevant data available, except 8 deviant for length of gestation by birthweight.

[a]Calculated on the basis of 4 calories/gm.

the rates of neonatal death among treatment groups diverged to the disadvantage of the Supplement group. The differences among the life tables, although at times verging on the 5% level, are not statistically significant at any stage of gestation. We are nevertheless faced with an unexpected and disturbing association of a high neonatal death rate with Supplement.

Characteristics of pregnancies ending in perinatal death. Data on individual neonatal deaths are given in Appendix 3.3. The mean duration of gestation among neonatal deaths in the Supplement group was 190 days, in the Complement group 199 days, and in the Control group 202 days. The mean birthweight in the Supplement group was 999 gm (including the twins), and no causes of death other than those associated with extreme prematurity were detected. Mean birthweight in the Complement group was 1,317 gm, and in the Control group 1,719 gm. While not statistically significant among this small number of cases, these large differences are suggestive of greater growth retardation among the deaths in the Supplement than in the other two groups.

Within the Supplement group, neonatal death was significantly associated with low Average Weight Gain ($r = -0.21$, $p < 0.001$). Other associations of interest, but not statistically significant, were with number of past low birthweight infants (r = 0.15); low Early Weight Gain (r = −0.13); somewhat high intake of beverage (r = 0.12); and with reduction in calories in the regular diet (r = −0.10).

The risk factors associated with fetal loss are of a different pattern from those associated with neonatal death. Fetal loss tended to be associated with social attributes of mothers that were antecedent to or independent of pregnancy, eg high maternal age, being out of school, higher occupational status of the mother's father, and lower average income per person in the household. There is very little overlap in characteristics associated with fetal and neonatal death, and the rates of fetal death are virtually identical in the three treatment groups. We consider therefore that these data on fetal deaths indicate no treatment effect, either adverse or beneficial.

Fetal Growth and Size at Birth

Fetal growth indices in this study are based on the dimensions of the infant at birth, particularly birthweight. These analyses take account of length of gestation, in order to separate small size owed to premature delivery from that owed to growth retardation. The results refer chiefly to the 768 singleton livebirths to mothers who remained active in the study to the time

TABLE 3.3. Duration of Gestation and Antecedent Maternal Factors

Maternal attributes	Supplement	Complement	Controls	Total
Past low birthweight[a] (n)	−.29**	−.05	.00	−.11*
Mother's education (no. years)	.15*	0.1	−.01	.05
On welfare vs others	−.15*	−.01	−.11	−.09**
At conception:				
Weight	.10	.07	.06	.08*
Ponderal index	.16*	.09	.06	.10**
At registration:				
Gestation	.12	.18**	−.04	.09*

Bivariate correlations within treatment groups among 805 women active to delivery (8 cases deviant for birthweight by gestation excluded). (Only variables with at least one significant association included.)

[a]Among multigravidae only.
*p < 0.05; **p < 0.01; ***p < 0.001.

TABLE 3.4. Treatment and Perinatal Deaths

		Fetal deaths			Neonatal deaths			
		gestation @ delivery (wks)			gestation @ delivery (wks)			
Treatment group	Births (n)	<20 weeks	≥20 weeks	Total (%)	<28	28–32	32–36	Total (%)
a) Twins as two births								
Supplement	267	3	8	11 (4.1)	6	3	1	10 (3.9)
Complement	274	4	9	13 (4.7)	3	2	1	6 (2.3)
Control	282	2	10	12 (4.3)	2	–	1	3 (1.1)
Total	823	9	27	36 (4.4)	11	5	3	19 (2.4)[a]
b) Twins excluded								
Supplement	259	3	7	10 (3.9)	4	3	1	8 (3.2)
Complement	270	4	9	13 (4.8)	1	1	1	3 (1.2)
Control	276	2	10	12 (4.3)	2	–	1	3 (1.1)
Total	805	9	26	35 (4.3)	7	4	3	14 (1.8)[b]

Numbers and percent of fetal and neonatal deaths among births to all participants active to delivery: a) each twin delivery counted as two births, b) twins excluded.

[a] Supplement vs all others, $\chi^2 = 3.59$, ns; Supplement vs Controls, $\chi^2 = 4.26$, $p < 0.05$.

[b] Supplement vs all others, $\chi^2 = 4.01$, $p < 0.05$; Supplement vs Controls $\chi^2 = 2.63$, ns.

TABLE 3.5. Fetal and Neonatal Mortality Compared

Maternal attributes	A. Fetal deaths				B. Neonatal deaths			
	Supp (n = 11)	Comp (n = 13)	Contr (n = 12)	Total (n = 36)	Supp (n = 9)	Comp (n = 5)	Contr (n = 3)	Total (n = 17)
Age	0.06	0.10	0.10	0.09*	0.05	−0.03	−0.15*	−0.03
Mothers occupational status (nonstudents)								
Occupational status maternal grandfather	0.05	0.18*	0.21**	0.15***				
On welfare	0.13*	−0.05	−0.08	0.00				
Student = 1, others = 0	−0.09	−0.11	−0.10	−0.10**				
Income/person (total family income)	−0.10	−0.10	−0.07	−0.09*				
	−0.01	−0.04	0.07	0.01				
At registration								
Gestation (days)	−0.18**	−0.14*	−0.11	−0.14***				
Triceps skinfold thickness	0.02	−0.06	0.12*	0.03				
Average, postregistration diet recalls:								
Beverage calories					0.12	0.10	—	0.12**
Beverage protein					0.12	0.08	—	0.10*
Count of cans					0.02	0.21**	—	0.11*
Urinary riboflavin (log of mean)					−0.04	−0.22**	—	−0.13**
Avg. no. cans/24 hr, health aide's history					0.03	0.14*	—	0.09
Early weight gain					−0.13	−0.02	−0.35***	−0.13***
Average weight gain					−0.21***	0.13*	−0.08	−0.07*

Correlations within treatment groups, a) fetal deaths with maternal attributes, b) neonatal deaths with maternal attributes of all 813 women active to delivery. (Only variables with at least one significant association included. Values are omitted where no correlations in a row are significant. The numbers included in each correlation coefficient vary slightly according to the availability of data.) Twins counted as one birth.
*p < 0.05; ** p < 0.01; ***p < 0.001.

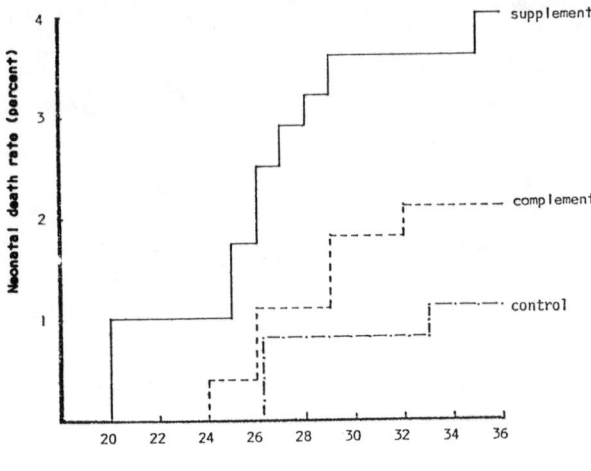

Fig. 3.2. Treatment and Neonatal Death. Cumulative rates of neonatal death (%) from life tables for each treatment group (see Appendix 3.2).

of delivery (birthweight was not recorded for one very premature infant who expired immediately at birth, and the case of Down syndrome was excluded from analysis, without knowledge of its treatment group or birthweight).

Birthweight and treatment (Table 3.6). The mean birthweight for the 768 births is shown in Table 3.6D. The mean birthweights were 2,938 gm for the Supplement group, 3,011 gm for the Complement group and 2,970 gm for the Control group. None of the differences between treatment groups was significant.* On the reasonable assumption that the one premature infant death of unknown weight and delivered at 197 days weighed 1,000 gm, the mean for the Supplement group would be reduced by 8 gm. This change would not have made the observed differences in mean birthweight between the Supplement group and the other two groups significant. The results also remain essentially unchanged with the inclusion in the analysis of women who did not sustain the regimen to delivery (Table 3.6C), or of women who delivered twins (Table 3.6B), or whose pregnancies terminated in fetal deaths with measured birthweight (Table 3.6A). There was, therefore,

*The outcome in terms of frequency of low birthweight (Table 3.11) is 18.5% for Supplement, 11.7% for Complement, and 16.3% for Controls. The crucial experimental comparisons of each treatment group against the Controls are not statistically significant, although the difference between Complement and the other two groups combined is significant when the unweighed Supplement premature is included.

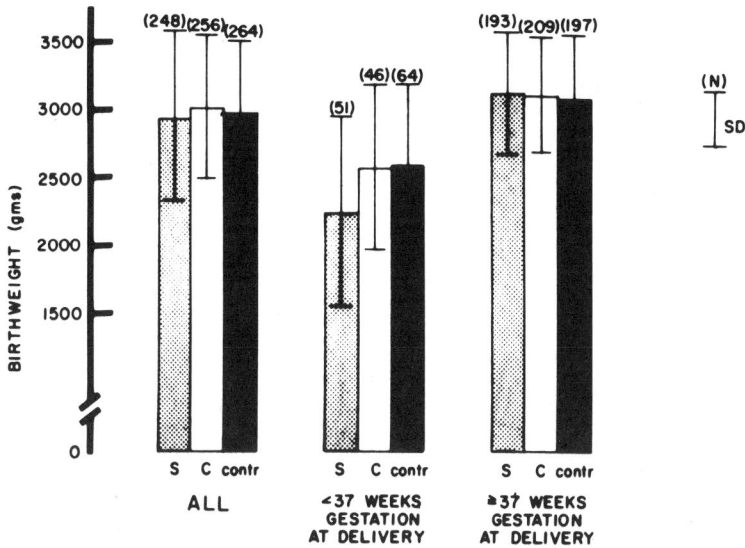

Fig. 3.3. Birthweight in Supplement (S), Complement (C), and Control (contr) groups among premature and mature deliveries.

no significant relationship of birthweight to nutritional supplementation.

Birthweight, treatment, and entry cohort (Table 3.7). We showed that the significant effect of the high protein Supplement on maternal weight gain was conditional on enrollment for prenatal care before 15 weeks gestation. In the present analysis of birthweight, we did not find analogous conditional effects for entry cohorts defined by stage of gestation. Thus, mean birthweight in the earliest entry cohort — in which Supplement increased weight gain — showed no effect of treatment. On the contrary, mean birthweight of the Supplement group in this cohort was 96 gm less than in the Control group. In later entry cohorts, in which Supplement did not affect maternal weight gain, the mean birthweight of the Supplement group was 20 gm heavier than that of the Control group.

Birthweight, treatment, and maturity (Table 3.8 and Fig. 3.3). The apparent increase in the number of very early deliveries in the Supplement group requires that we determine the degree and the manner in which length of gestation mediates birthweight. To do so we analyzed mature and premature deliveries separately. Among infants born mature (37 weeks gestation or later), no significant differences in birthweight were observed among treatment groups, although the two supplemented groups were at a slight advantage. The means for the three treatment groups were 3,112; 3,103, and 3,088 gm for the Supplement, Complement, and Control groups respectively.

Among infants born prematurely, Supplement produced growth retardation. Birthweight was significantly lower in the Supplement group: for deliveries under 37 weeks, means were 2,254, 2,577, and 2,587 gm for the Supplement, Complement, and Control groups respectively (see Table 3.9) (Supplement vs Controls, $t = 2.83$, $p < 0.01$; Supplement vs Complement, $t = 2.45$, $p < 0.02$). The appearance of growth retardation could have been produced by the maldistribution of Supplement cases among very early prematures. Depressed birthweight in the Supplement group was present, however, in infants delivered in each two week interval of gestation up to 37 weeks (Table 3.8).

When the 8 cases with birthweight more than 3 standard deviations from expectation for their given length of gestation (calculated from first day of last menstrual period) are included in the analysis,* the birthweights of the prematures of the Supplement group remain significantly low.

Birthweight, maturity, and entry cohort (Table 3.9). Among infants born *mature*, mean birthweight was not significantly related to treatment in any cohort. Among infants born *premature*, mean birthweight was lower in the Supplement group than in the Complement group in all 4 entry cohorts, and in 3 of the 4 it was lower than in the Control group. The deficit in birthweight in the Supplement group compared with the other 2 treatment groups, however, was more marked among women in whom nutritional supplementation was begun at an early stage in pregnancy. For the 2 earliest entry cohorts combined (< 20 weeks gestation) that delivered prematurely in the Supplement group, the deficit as compared with Controls was signifi-

---

*In Table 3.6E and in all subsequent tables that require the use of duration of gestation, we have excluded 8 cases in which birthweight was more than 3 standard deviations beyond that expected for the recorded gestation. This procedure, derived from the analyses of Milner and Richards (1974), is an attempt to correct for the grosser mis-estimates of gestational length which sometimes occur.

cant at the p <0.001 level. This deficit among the early entry cohorts is reminiscent of the depressing effect of Supplement on later maternal weight gain among women who entered the study before 15 weeks gestation and who delivered prematurely.

There was no effect of Supplement on maternal weight gain in any of the cohorts recruited after 15 weeks, however, in contrast with its depressing effect on the birthweight of prematures in these cohorts.

Treatment effects on newborn dimensions (Table 3.10). None of the dimensions of infants at birth was significantly related to nutritional supplementation. For the subsample of singleton livebirths, the only statistically significant effect, and that not a strong one, is on length of gestation for the Complement group. Analysis of relationships controlled for length of gestation revealed that the small advantage in birthweight in the Complement group can be accounted for by the increased length of gestation in that group.

Dietary indices and newborn dimensions. Since treatment group assignment produced no significant beneficial effects on newborn dimensions, we deemed it important to test the quality of the data. We therefore explored a large number of relationships between newborn dimensions and indices connected with nutrition. The correlations shown in Appendix 3.4 are bivariate. Partial correlations controlled for length of gestation make no material difference to the relationships.

In the *total* study population (that is, all treatment groups combined) nearly all relationships involving maternal weight gain and newborn size were as anticipated. Maternal weight gain relates to newborn dimensions in a fairly consistent and expected manner. Thus, relationships with birthweight and with placental weight are strong, those with length and head circumference less so.

Within treatment groups, however, the pattern of correlations differs sharply. Here we should perhaps observe that by virtue of the study design, treatment effects can be measured against departures in either direction, by either or both of the supplemented groups, from the norms of the Control group. With regard to maternal weight gain, for

TABLE 3.6. Mean Birthweight by Treatment Group in Variously Defined Experimental Groups

A. 864 singletons and 18 twin *total births* to 873 women assigned to treatment groups who remained eligible for inclusion in the study up to delivery, yielding 831 singletons and 16 twins of known birthweight. (Birthweight was unknown in 7 of 9 early fetal deaths, in 15 of 27 late fetal deaths, in one singleton neonatal death of 197 days gestation, and in one twin neonatal death.)

B. 818 singleton and 17 twin livebirths to 827 women who remained eligible for inclusion in the study up to delivery, yielding 833 of known birthweight. (Birthweight was unknown in one singleton and one twin neonatal death.)

C. 818 *singleton livebirths* to women who remained eligible for inclusion in the study up to delivery [including 48 who chose to discontinue supplements and for whom birthweight was known] yielding 817 of known birthweight. (Birthweight was unknown in one neonatal death.)

D. 768 *singleton livebirths* of known birthweight *active to delivery*, excluding 48 whose mothers chose to discontinue supplements, and one Down syndrome infant.

E. 760 *singleton livebirths* of known birthweight *active to delivery*, excluding one Down syndrome infant, and 8 cases deviant for length of gestation by birthweight.

| | Treatment group | | | |
Sample	Supplement	Complement	Controls	Total
A n = 847	2,894 ± 657 (276)	2,980 ± 604 (298)	2,928 ± 756 (273)	2,935 ± 614 (847)
B n = 833	2,912 ± 631 (273)	3,001 ± 556 (291)	2,948 ± 548 (269)	2,954 ± 580 (833)
C n = 817	2,936 ± 606 (266)	3,028 ± 569 (287)	2,967 ± 535 (264)	2,978 ± 552 (817)
D n = 768	2,938 ± 611 (248)	3,011 ± 508 (256)	2,970 ± 535 (264)	2,972 ± 553 (768)
E n = 760	2,933 ± 614 (244)	3,008 ± 500 (255)	2,961 ± 535 (261)	2,968 ± 554 (760)

instance, we conclude that a treatment effect resides in the Complement group. This conclusion follows because maternal weight gain relates to newborn dimensions strongly in the Control group as well as in the Supplement group, but weakly, if at all, in the Complement group. Similarly with weight gain from conception until recruitment into the study, the correlations of newborn dimensions exhibit the same singularity in the Complement group. Thus, within the Supplement and Control groups, but not within the Complement group, newborn dimensions correlate positively with the mother's weight gain before recruitment.

The conclusion that there was a treatment effect in the Complement group is also compatible with the contrasting pattern of correlations of reported diet intake with newborn dimensions. With these correlations the arrangement of the treatment groups is reversed. Dietary intake indices relate significantly to newborn dimensions in the Complement group, and in that group alone.

Control variables and conditional effects. When the several maternal characteristics that are significantly related to birth weight were controlled by multiple regression analysis (Appendices 3.5a–e) the effect of treatment on birthweight was little altered. The result held whether length of gestation was considered as an outcome and omitted or considered as a control variable and entered in the equation. Thus, the absence of a favorable treatment effect cannot be attributed to the maldistribution of potentially confounding variables.

From the multiple regression analysis we note the following:

3.5a: This analysis controls for the criteria used in selection and stratification of the sample, and also for parity and smoking. Controlling for these variables reduces the deficit in birthweight between the Supplement and Control groups to 14 gm, while the Complement group's advantage over Controls rises to 56 gm.

3.5b: When duration of gestation at delivery is included in the analysis and thus controlled, the mean for birthweight in the Supplement group was 39 gm less than Controls, and in the Complement group 3 gm less than Controls.

TABLE 3.7. Birthweight, Treatment, and Entry Cohort

Entry cohort (weeks of gestation)	Treatment group			
	Supplement	Complement	Control	Total
<15	2,962 ± 623 (81)	3,012 ± 550 (98)	3,058 ± 491 (110)	3,016 ± 552 (289)
15–19	2,877 ± 672 (68)	3,036 ± 428 (59)	2,959 ± 503 (68)	2,954 ± 553 (195)
20–24	3,012 ± 585 (54)	2,987 ± 535 (60)	2,787 ± 647 (49)	2,935 ± 595 (163)
25+	2,863 ± 507 (41)	2,987 ± 458 (38)	2,934 ± 494 (34)	2,926 ± 490 (113)
All	2,938 ± 611 (248)[a]	3,011 ± 508 (256)[a]	2,970 ± 535 (264)[a]	2,973 ± 553 (768)[a]

Mean birthweight in grams (± SD) among liveborn singletons (numbers in parentheses) by treatment group and entry cohort defined by stage of gestation at enrollment.

[a] 8 cases with birthweight 3 SD from the mean for length of gestation included only in total row (4 Supplement, 1 Complement, 3 Control.)

TABLE 3.8. Birthweight, Treatment, and Maturity

Treatment group	Gestation at delivery (weeks)					
	−30	31–32	33–34	35–36	37+	Total
Supplement	1,293 ± 455 (9)	1,979 ± 411 (5)	2,224 ± 293 (13)	2,688 ± 528 (24)	3,112 ± 447 (193)	2,938 ± 611 (248)[a]
Complement	1,588 ± 827 (5)	2,410 ± 522 (4)	2,469 ± 355 (14)	2,886 ± 385 (23)	3,103 ± 427 (209)	3,011 ± 508 (256)[a]
Control	1,528 ± 546 (5)	2,824 ± 133 (4)	2,515 ± 510 (24)	2,782 ± 398 (31)	3,088 ± 459 (197)	2,970 ± 535 (264)[a]
Total	1,432 ± 612 (19)	2,372 ± 526 (13)	2,428 ± 474 (51)	2,784 ± 446 (78)	3,101 ± ( ) (599)	2,973 ± 553 (768)[a]

Mean birthweight in grams (± SD) among liveborn singletons (numbers in parentheses) by treatment group and length of gestation at delivery.

[a] 8 cases with birthweight 3 SD from the mean for length of gestation (4 Supplement, 1 Complement, 3 Control) omitted from all but Total column.

3.5c: There was a significant interaction between treatment with Supplement and cigarette smoking: Supplement and, to a lesser extent, Complement protected against the effects of cigarette smoking on birthweight (see below). The interaction between treatment with Supplement and number of past low birthweight infants was not significant, but still striking: for each past low birthweight delivery, birthweight was on average 161 gm lower in the Supplement group than in the Control group. In the Complement group the comparable deficit was 112 gm.

3.5d: The interactions in Appendix 3.5c are much attenuated when length of gestation is controlled; hence, we conclude that in large part these interactions were mediated by length of gestation.

3.5e: Average daily calorie intake was significantly related to birthweight. The relationship was intensified after controlling for protein intake and for duration of gestation. Thus, the effect appears to be on fetal growth rate, rather than on duration of gestation, and to be accentuated by taking into account the balance between calorie and protein intake. Controlling for calorie intake, birthweight *decreased* with increased protein intake.

Two of the conditional effects found above deserve elaboration.

Newborn dimensions and smoking. Smoking was significantly related to newborn size in our data, as expected from many previously reported studies. We have reported elsewhere that in the Control group depressed maternal weight gain can account for three-quarters of the deficit in birthweight associated with smoking [Rush, 1974]. The implication of this finding is that *heavy smoking* has nutritional effects during gestation. The deficit in birthweight among the infants of heavy smokers as compared with nonsmokers in the Control group disappeared among infants of heavy smokers as compared with nonsmokers in the supplemented groups. (Fig. 3.4). Among smokers the difference in birthweight between Controls and the supplemented groups was highly significant. Increased length of

TABLE 3.9. Birthweight, Treatment, Maturity, and Stage of Gestation at Entry[a]

Maturity	Entry cohort	Supplement	Complement	Controls	Total
Delivered < 37 weeks	<15	2,150 ± 637 (15)	2,440 ± 624 (20)	2,590 ± 614 (20)	2,415 ± 648 (55)
	15-19	2,292 ± 784 (18)	3,048 ± 529 (6)	2,857 ± 406 (22)	2,661 ± 669 (46)
	20-24	2,180 ± 689 (9)	2,473 ± 566 (11)	2,110 ± 608 (13)	2,250 ± 638 (33)
	25+	2,425 ± 450 (9)	2,693 ± 483 (9)	2,607 ± 314 (9)	2,575 ± 437 (27)
	All	2,254* ± 682 (51)	2,577* ± 609 (46)	2,587* ± 579 (64)	2,478 ± 640 (161)
Delivered ≥ 37 weeks	<15	3,146 ± 448 (66)	3,160 ± 417 (78)	3,162 ± 389 (90)	3,157 ± 416 (234)
	15-19	3,087 ± 475 (50)	3,035 ± 415 (53)	3,008 ± 536 (46)	3,044 ± 476 (149)
	20-24	3,178 ± 388 (45)	3,102 ± 453 (49)	3,031 ± 459 (36)	3,109 ± 437 (130)
	25+	2,987 ± 451 (32)	3,078 ± 409 (29)	3,052 ± 494 (25)	3,037 ± 452 (86)
	All	3,112 ± 447 (193)	3,103 ± 427 (209)	3,088 ± 459 (197)	3,101 ± 444 (599)

Mean birthweight in grams (± SD) among liveborn singletons (numbers in parentheses) by treatment group, entry cohort defined by stage of gestation at registration, and prematurity.

[a] 8 cases deviant for length of gestation versus birthweight omitted.

*Supplement vs Controls, t = 2.83, p < 0.01.
Supplement vs Complement, t = 2.45, p < 0.02.

TABLE 3.10. Treatment Effects on Selected Newborn Dimensions

Newborn dimensions	Supplement	Complement[b]	Controls
Birthweight (n = 769)	−0.05	0.05	−0.01
Length (n = 709)	−0.01	0.05	−0.04
Ponderal index (n = 708)	−0.02	0.00	0.02
Head circumference (n = 703)	0.01	0.04	−0.05
Placental weight (n = 577)	0.02	−0.01	−0.01
Arm girths (n = 676)	−0.01	0.06	−0.04
Subscapular skinfold (n = 674)	−0.01	0.02	−0.01
Triceps skinfold (n = 675)	−0.01	0.03	−0.02
Length of gestation[a] (n = 760)	−0.02	0.07*	−0.05

Bivariate correlations of newborn dimensions and treatment group assignment among 769 liveborn singletons. All these relationships remained insignificant when the effect of gestation was partialled out.

[a] 8 cases with birthweight deviant for length of gestation omitted.
[b] Down syndrome infant included.
*$p < 0.05$.

gestation accounted for part of this effect of supplementation. Supplementation evidently protected both against premature delivery and growth retardation.

Newborn dimensions and past low birthweight. In the total study population, we found (as expected) that women who had previously been delivered of low birthweight infants tended to have infants of lower birthweight than other women. This risk was exacerbated in the Supplement group. Curtailed gestation is clearly the factor responsible for low birthweight in these cases. Birthweight, length, head circumference, and placental weight were all similarly affected. Ponderal index was unaffected, that is, the infants were proportionately small in all dimensions, as would be expected with prematurity, but not with growth retardation.

Women on Supplement who reported past low birthweight deliveries had a large proportion of neonatal deaths (3 of 31 or 97/1,000) as well as an excess of prematures. These women reported a degree of adherence to the nutritional regimen no different from the rest of the Supplement group. Nor was the noxious effect of Supplement in this subgroup mediated to any notable degree by depressed maternal weight gain.

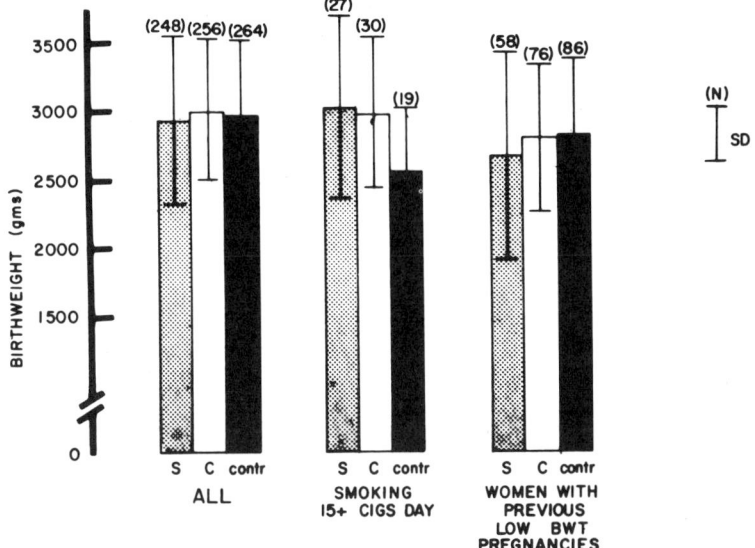

Fig. 3.4. Birthweight in Supplement (S), Complement (C), and Control (contr) groups among women who were smokers, and among women with previous deliveries of low birthweight infants.

DISCUSSION

Between-Group Differences: Outcome

Differences in mean birthweight among the three randomly assigned treatment groups were not statistically significant. The preconditions for testing the central hypothesis gave a chance of detecting a significant difference 4 out of 5 times. The null hypothesis was that nutritional supplementation would not produce a change in mean birthweight of 125 gm in either direction more than 1 in 20 times. For the total study group this hypothesis must be accepted.

Mean birthweight did not reflect the increment in maternal weight gain among women recruited early in pregnancy that was produced by the high protein Supplement and reported in Chapter 2. This dissociation of the effect of the high protein Supplement on maternal weight gain from its effects on fetal growth was contrary to our hypothesis, and unexpected in view of the strong relation of maternal weight gain and birthweight found in many studies, including this one.

TABLE 3.11. Summary of Results by Treatment Group

	Supplement	Complement	Control
Calorie intake/day during study			
Total	2,326 ± 764	2,272 ± 773	2,065 ± 699
Beverage only	326 ± 157	233 ± 118	
Without beverage	2,000 ± 739	2,039 ± 760	
n	231	234	249
Protein intake/day (gm) during study			
Total	101.9 ± 32.4	82.7 ± 31.2	79.3 ± 29.3
Beverage only	27.7 ± 13.3	4.5 ± 2.6	
Without beverage	74.2 ± 28.0	78.2 ± 30.9	
n	229	234	248
% calories as protein	~17.5	~14.6	~15.4
Weight gain (lbs/wk)			
Early	0.99*b ± 0.66 (211)	0.89 ± 0.71 (212)	0.85 ± 0.77 (225)
Average	0.96 ± 0.50 (240)	0.95 ± 0.44 (245)	0.91 ± 0.45 (255)
Correlation with calorie intake			
Early Weight Gain (with early calories)	0.04	0.07	0.17*
Average Weight Gain (with avg calories)	0.13	0.08	0.07**

Length of gestation, (total active population) by life table analysis			
% <20 wks	2.8	3.6	0.6
% <25 wks	4.6	4.3	3.2
% <30 wks	9.2	5.7	4.7
% <33 wks	11.9	8.3	6.8
% <35 wks	16.4	13.9	15.2
% <37 wks	24.8	21.8	26.0
Birthweight (liveborn singletons)			
Mean (gm)	2,938 ± 611 (248)	3,011 ± 508 (256)	2,967 ± 535 (264)
% < 2,500 gm	18.5 (249)	11.7*a (256)	16.3 (264)
Correlations with:			
Average daily calories	0.06	0.13*	0.02
Early Weight Gain	0.19**	0.13	0.24***
Average Weight Gain	0.33***	0.15*	0.26***
No. cigarettes/day	−0.05	−0.12*	−0.24***
No. past low birthweight infants	−0.32***	−0.23**	−0.20*
Neonatal deaths			
% of Total livebirths	3.9	2.3	1.1
Correlation with:			
Past low birthweight (n)	0.15	0.08	0.05
Gestation at registration	−0.04	−0.04	0.08
Early Weight Gain	−0.13	0.02	−0.35***
Average Weight Gain	−0.21***	0.13*	−0.08

*p < .05.
**p < .01.
***p < .001.
a vs other 2 groups combined.
b vs controls.

We studied premature and mature deliveries separately. Among mature births, mean birthweight was slightly higher in both supplemented groups — 24 gm in favor of Supplement and 15 gm in favor of Complement. Among the prematures, we were startled to find significantly lower mean birthweight in the Supplement group than in either the Complement or the Control group. At each interval of gestation below 37 weeks, mean birthweight was lower in the Supplement group. The high protein Supplement evidently retarded fetal growth.

Within-Group Differences: Process

We leave aside for the moment discussion of this adverse effect, and consider effects seen *within* treatment groups. By the logic of the double-blind nutritional intervention, differences between the supplemented groups can be attributed to differences in the content of the supplements, and the size of the effect can be measured against the Control group. Differences from the Control group that are equal for the two supplemented groups can probably also be attributed to the content of the supplements, although with less certainty. In such a case the penumbra of activity connected with the intervention that differentiates both supplemented groups from the Control group can be neither neutralized nor dismissed. When differences among the three treatment groups occur in a gradient, interpretation depends on the pattern found.

In the case of birthweight, associations with reported diet intake were almost entirely accounted for by the Complement group. Similar associations were obtained for head circumference, and for ponderal index, although not for length. Surprisingly, these conditional treatment effects in the Complement group linked diet intake to newborn dimensions *without* the mediation of maternal weight gain. The associations of birthweight and the other newborn dimensions with maternal weight gain were weakest in the Complement group. In contrast, as we had anticipated, they were strong in the Supplement and Control groups.

With Complement, therefore, one may argue that diet intake was transmuted into fetal growth. This occurred without Complement having accelerated maternal weight gain, which in turn is consistent with the observation that maternal weight gain in the Complement group bore little relationship to fetal dimensions. Any explanation of the pattern of association among the three treatment groups surely requires that the metabolic pathways of the ingested nutrients were differently influenced by the content of the two dietary supplements. We know that the high protein Supplement, in contrast with the balanced Complement, did produce an increment in maternal weight gain. This increment in the Supplement group was *not* transmuted into fetal growth. The conversion failed to occur, as indicated by the lack of correlation of newborn dimensions with diet intake, despite the fact that newborn dimensions were correlated as expected with maternal weight gain.

It can be seen that *in the total population* of births the variables supposedly connected with the processes of fetal growth relate with measures of diet intake in the direction anticipated from our hypotheses. Contrary to these same hypotheses, however, outcomes at birth *within treatment groups* do not relate to the assignment to the experimental nutritional treatment. Neither treatment with Supplement nor with Complement (when compared with either or both of the other two groups), nor the amount of supplementary beverage taken (when compared within each of the treatment groups), significantly increased measures of size at birth.

Nonetheless, we conclude that assignment to the Complement group potentiated an association of regular diet with fetal growth. Complement appears to have allowed nutrients to be channeled directly to the fetus and to bypass maternal stores. This interpretation is compatible both with the absence of an effect on weight gain in the Complement group, and with certain placental biochemical and chemical effects observed but not as yet reported except in a doctoral dissertation [Pereira, 1977].

Although the fact or the amount of Complement treatment had no detectable effect on fetal growth as measured by newborn dimensions, we must allow that an effect too small to detect at the level of our test may have been present. Low birthweight was least frequent with Complement, verging on statistical significance. The difference in birthweight between the Complement and Control groups in this study was 41 gm. With a large array of variables controlled in a multiple regression analysis, the adjusted difference was 56 gm. The size of this difference is consistent with a number of results in other studies, as we shall discuss in Chapter V. With hindsight, we now see that to set the gain expected in our study at 125 gm was optimistic, even had the target population been unequivocally and chronically malnourished.

Conditional beneficial effects among women who entered treatment early were not found for birthweight as they had been for maternal weight gain. Three other conditional treatment effects on birthweight were found, however. One effect was in a favorable direction: both nutritional treatments appear to have protected against the deficits in birthweight caused by heavy smoking. The other two effects were in an unfavorable direction: the infants born prematurely to women who had entered treatment early in the high protein Supplement group suffered greater deficits in birthweight than those born to women who entered treatment later. and women with a history of previous low birthweight in particular were adversely affected by the high protein Supplement.

Adverse effects of the high protein Supplement. The women on the high protein Supplement suffered an excess of early premature deliveries (under 30 weeks gestation) and a consequent excess of neonatal deaths, as well as intrauterine growth retardation at all stages of prematurity. Numbers were small, but the nearly two-fold risk of delivery before 30 weeks gestation in the Supplement group was on the verge of statistical significance, and the lower mean birthweight among Supplement group prematures was highly significant.

The entire excess of neonatal deaths in the Supplement group was located among the extremely early premature. After 30 weeks gestation there was but one death in each treatment group was located among the extremely early prematures. After the Supplement group infants who died in the newborn period were probably growth retarded, this point cannot be securely established for lack of comparison with surviving infants in other treatment groups of the same gestational age.

The relationships of prematurity with these outcomes, with maternal weight gain, and with other characteristics of the pregnancies lends credence to a causal sequence initiated by treatment with the high protein Supplement. The distinctiveness of the pattern of associations among these adverse outcomes is emphasized by the divergence among neonatal and fetal deaths. Neonatal deaths were connected with treatment group, and other associated factors were mainly biological and nutritional and related to current pregnancy. Fetal deaths were unconnected with treatment group, and other associated factors were mainly social and antecedent to pregnancy.

Since all Supplement neonatal deaths occurred among premature births, it is not unexpected that associations of neonatal deaths were of a kind with those of prematurity. Both neonatal death and prematurity were associated with past delivery of low birthweight infants, with thinness at conception, and with good adherence to the treatment regimen. With death or prematurity Supplement intake was higher than with term births, but regular diet was cut back beyond the extra calories supplied by Supplement. The pattern of weight gain was similar too. The group of mothers adversely affected tended to have entered treatment early in pregnancy, to have gained weight well at the onset, and to have lost their advantage in weight gain later in pregnancy. Mothers' education and early entry into treatment were also associated with adverse outcome. These two variables can be seen as behavioral indicators; the associations conform both with reported high complicance with the treatment regimen, and with the Early Weight Gain among these women.

One must consider whether the adverse effects might not have occurred among all women on Supplement, but that they recovered if their pregnancies survived the second trimester. A close examination of the data on maternal weight gain does not support this hypothesis. Thus, we found no evidence of a midpregnancy deceleration of weight gain among any group of women excepting those on Supplement who delivered prematurely. On the other hand, the data do suggest — although they do not fully establish — that those who had borne past low birthweight infants and those who were thin at conception were at greater risk than other women.

The pattern of associations among adverse outcomes in the Supplement group renders an attribution to chance unlikely. Hypotheses that we have entertained to explain the findings include a) toxic effects of a contaminant; b) an overloading effect intrinsic to the protein (casein) of the Supplement or, less likely, to other components; c) an anorectic effect of the high protein diet on maternal appetite and hence on birthweight.

A toxic contaminant is improbable. A toxin seems unlikely to be selective of such biological characteristics as number of past low birthweight infants and weight at conception, nor would one anticipate recovery in late pregnancy from a dose steadily accumulating thoughout pregnancy. There was no suggestion that the effects of the Supplement differed among the batches of beverage manufactured for the study at different periods.

An overloading effect of high protein, while not incompatible with midpregnancy manifestations and subsequent recovery for most, is certainly compatible with a vulnerable group who have had difficulty in adapting to and assimilating an unaccustomed high dose of protein. An anorectic action of high protein intake on appetite is also compatible with effects limited to a vulnerable group of women. The sequence of events is consistent with the following:

1. Early in treatment: high level adherence to beverage regimen leads to high Early Weight Gain. 2. Later in treatment: high level adherence to beverage leads to anorexia from high protein intake, with consequent reduced caloric intake and weight gain, and retardation of fetal growth. 3. Finally: some combination of the above factors leading to markedly premature delivery.

The chain of events is surely close to that laid out, but an indirect effect of high protein intake on appetite seems by itself insufficient to account for the results. This we infer from the size of such effects as can be attributed solely to the level of diet intake, as seen in this and other studies. The intrinsic quality of the Supplement itself is thus brought into question.

CONCLUSION

In conclusion, in this trial of prenatal nutritional supplementation the only statistically significant favorable effect on the main outcome criterion was the prevention of depressed birthweight among the offspring of supplemented mothers who smoked heavily. On the subsidiary outcome criterion of length of gestation, the balanced calorie/protein Complement also had a significantly favorable effect, but one insufficient to produce a significant effect on birthweight. The absence of main effects cannot reasonably be attributed to nonadherence to the regimen, given the battery of data reported in an earlier chapter devoted to this question. Those data indicated quite satisfactory adherence. We have seen too, that adherence was sufficient to cause significant adverse effects among a minority of women exposed to the high protein Supplement.

It is clear to us that a number of our preconceived notions about maternal nutrition and fetal growth must be abandoned. To help explain the absence of discernible favorable effects on fetal growth, we would draw attention to previous observations on the threshold levels of prenatal nutrition and on the size of effects to be expected. In the Dutch famine study, effects of nutritional deprivation on newborn size were found only below a threshold level of food rations [Stein et al, 1975]. In our study population, protein intake met recommended levels, although calorie intake was somewhat low. Above a threshold level, we presume that the greater part of the association of regular diet with newborn size is not causal but the common consequence of maternal size. Thomson [1959] likewise interpreted his data in these terms. Yet in our study, unlike Thomson's, maternal size did not account for the whole of the association of diet with birthweight. Thus some room for a dietary effect may have remained which our design was too weak to detect.

With regard to the adverse effect of the high protein Supplement, our results, we believe, give a warning that must be heeded. The metabolic pathways as well as the ultimate effects of the high protein and the balanced supplements were evidently different. In the study initiated by Bacon Chow in Taiwan, 83 women supplemented with 40 gm of protein and 800 calories did rather better than controls, although not significantly so [Herriot, Hsueh, Aitchison, 1978]. These women may have been protected by the high intake of carbohydrate that accompanied the protein.

Animal observations also indicate that a high protein diet given to unaccustomed subjects may have untoward results. Thus in a study of protein-deprived rhesus monkeys a protein diet of 4 gm/kg body weight, but not diets of 1 and 2 gm/kg, led to accelerated maternal weight gain. This weight gain was not translated into birthweight. Further, gestation was significantly shortened in the group on the high protein diet [Riopelle, Hale, Watts, 1976; Riopelle and Favrett, 1977]. All three of these findings are consistent with our study, although the analogy is not perfect. For instance, among the rhesus monkeys on the higher protein diet, no evidence presented indicated that there is a vulnerable group with a deficit in birthweight and high neonatal mortality, and fetal mortality was highest among the protein deprived. Nonetheless, the resemblances of the results in the primate study and in ours are striking enough to give us pause.

Our study, like a number of others, was begun when protein was commonly assumed to be deficient in the diets of the poor, and to constitute a limiting nutrient. The results of our studies seem to us to require that a hold be put on high protein supplementary food programs among pregnant women. In Guatemala, the apparent increment in birthweight attributed to a protein-free supplement was not less than that attributed to a supplement containing protein [Habicht et al, 1974]. It should be noted that the level of protein in the Guatemalan supplement was much less than the level in our study. Thus the Guatemalan study does not speak to the likelihood of adverse effects of high protein supplements.* At the same time it does not point to any advantage of moderate protein supplements. This must be a time for reflection and further research.

SUMMARY

The outcome at birth of a randomized controlled trial of prenatal nutritional supplementation is reported with respect to duration of gestation, perinatal mortaility, and infant size at birth. Birthweight was the main outcome criterion around which the study was designed. The only significant favorable effect on birthweight was the prevention of depressed birthweight among the offspring of supplemented mothers who smoked heavily. On the subsidiary outcome criterion of length of gestation, the balanced calorie/protein Complement had a significant if slight favorable effect. An additional treatment effect presumed to be favorable is seen in the strengthened correlation between diet intake and fetal growth in the treatment group on balanced protein/calorie supplementation. This finding presumably indicates facilitation of nutrient supplies to the fetus. With high protein supplementation, the only effects recognized were adverse, apart from that with smoking. There was an excess of very early prematures and an excess of associated neonatal deaths, both on the verge of statistical significance; further, there was significant growth retardation among deliveries up to 37 weeks gestation. These adverse effects seem likely to be owed to the intrinsic properties of the high protein Supplement, and it is proposed that a hold be put on high protein supplementation of pregnant women. The differences in the effects of high protein and balanced supplementation need further study.

---

*Further on this point, infants with unknown birthweight who are likely to include many prematures were excluded from the published analyses; the prematurely born were excluded from most analyses, and never reported on separately. Moreover, effects on gestation have not been reported.

Chapter IV

Outcome at One Year of Age: Effects on Somatic and Psychological Measures

In this chapter we analyze the outcome of the randomized controlled trial of prenatal nutritional supplementation in infants around one year of age. The outcomes reported are somatic and psychological measures of development.

At the outset of the trial, we postulated two alternative pathways through which nutritional effects on later mental function might be mediated. The first was through intrauterine growth.

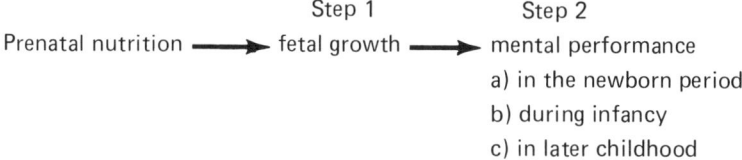

```
                        Step 1           Step 2
Prenatal nutrition ——▶ fetal growth ——▶ mental performance
                                         a) in the newborn period
                                         b) during infancy
                                         c) in later childhood
```

The existence of such a pathway was supported by some of the human studies linking birthweight with cognitive performance in childhood [Wiener, 1970; Drillien, 1972]. Results of such studies have not been consistent and in many, the relationships have been nonexistent or weak [Douglas, 1960; Record, McKeown, and Edwards, 1969a]. We ourselves failed to confirm the existence of such a pathway in our study of young adult survivors of the Dutch famine of 1944–45 [Stein et al, 1975]. In that case, severe prenatal undernutrition produced intrauterine growth retardation (Step 1 in the pathway), yet the generation of young men who survived prenatal famine exposure seemed in no way handicapped in terms of cognitive performance. The result cast doubt on the validity of Step 2 of the pathway. The possibility could

---

*Nathan Brody is a co-author of this chapter.

not be ruled out that effects on mental function did occur, however, but either were confined to the early years of life, or impinged on unmeasured functions.

The second postulated pathway was direct, and not mediated by fetal growth; in this causal model, prenatal nutrition affects mental performance independently of any effect on fetal growth.

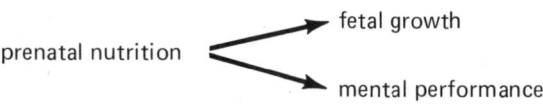

We know, from the results reported in Chapter III, that in the present study supplementation did not significantly accelerate fetal growth in the study population as a whole. Hence the overall outcomes at one year can provide a test only of the second causal model. Although the existence of such a direct pathway from prenatal nutrition to cognitive function was also not confirmed in our study of the Dutch famine, effects cannot be ruled out for the same reasons as indicated for the first pathway. Again, effects may have been confined to the early years of life, or impinged on unmeasured functions.

METHODS AND PROCEDURES

We showed in the first chapter the retention of subjects in the trial from the time when women were identified as eligible for recruitment (1,255 women) until birth and neonatal survival of their offspring (755 singletons and 12 twins). The present report concerns the 633 (84%) surviving singleton infants examined in the study around one year of age. Twins, although examined, are omitted from the analysis. Losses to the study sample between the newborn period and one year of age, as with losses at earlier stages, did not occur selectively in one or other treatment group.

We therefore proceed, confident that randomization was effective, that the assigned treatments were followed, and that a representative series of survivors was retained for our study. We can be less confident that the number of subjects is sufficient to test the effect of supplementation on any one particular measure. The numbers recruited into the trial were determined from the requirements for detecting a rise of 125 gms in birthweight (α = 0.05 on a two-tailed test, β = 0.02), and not from those for detecting effects at one year of age. No criteria for predicting the magnitude of effects that might follow prenatal nutritional supplementation were available to us.

The numbers subjected to each test varied (Tables 4.1 and 4.2). The chief reason for these differences in numbers was that some of the psychological measures (the object–permanence test, the measures based on play, and the visual habituation measures) were added after the study was under way. A less practical reason was an inability to test some infants, either for some or all procedures. During the testing session the Bayley tests were administered first. Some children became fussy or uncooperative during testing and did not always continue the session to completion. We did not invariably succeed in scheduling a repeat visit. As the table shows, losses for any test were not significantly different among the three treatment groups.

Mothers were invited to attend when the children reached the age of 44 weeks (308–315 days). In fact, because of delays in attendance and scheduling (especially with mothers who had left the New York area), the mean age of the children at the time of testing is 351 days (±48), with the distribution skewed to older ages.

Testing Procedures

Children were brought by appointment to the research center, accompanied by their mothers or guardians. They spent a whole morning or afternoon with the investigative team, in a relaxed atmosphere (with frequent rest periods and juice and crackers offered between examinations). The psychological measures were obtained first, followed by the somatic measures. Few children were upset by the procedures. Whenever either the psychological or the somatic findings pointed up problems, appropriate referrals were arranged. The psychological tests and somatic measurements were carried out by doctoral candidates with Master's degrees in psychology. Training sessions were held, and an acceptable degree of interrater reliability was achieved, varying somewhat by the measure.

The *somatic* measures reported include height, weight, head circumference, arm girth, and triceps and subscapular skinfold thickness, all obtained by standard techniques. The *psychological* measures reported include the Bayley Scales of Infant Development (Mental and Motor Scales), and a test of object-permanence [Corman and Escalona, 1969]. For each of these, the standard procedure for administration and scoring was followed. Raw scores were preferred to scaled scores for the Bayley tests. Two other less familiar testing situations, one involving free play and the other visual habituation, were adapted for the study.

Play was observed through one-way mirrors. The child was placed in a rectangular room (1.83 m × 4.27 m) divided by tape on the floor into nine rectangular areas. Eight of the nine rectangles each contained a different toy. The mother was seated in the ninth rectangle in a chair at the end of the room with the child on the floor beside her. Observers used event recorders to note the child's movement away from the mother and from one rectangle to another. They also recorded the frequency and the duration in seconds of each episode of toy play. An episode was defined as a discrete phase of continuous involvement with a particular toy or combination of toys. In addition, each episode of play was assigned a scaled score for degree of sophistication, using as a basis the Uzgiris-Hunt measure of development of schema in relation to objects. This scale of "sophistication of play" is assumed to represent a developmental sequence in which certain modes of interaction with objects occur prior to others. The score assigned to a child was the median for all episodes of play. In all, five measures of play behavior were derived: interval before the child began play (latency period); number of rectangles entered; number of play episodes; mean duration of play episodes; and sophistication of play.

Visual habituation was tested with the child seated in the mother's lap and placed 1.22 m from a light panel. Twelve colored lights arranged in a masonite board in the pattern of a cross constituted the stimulus display. The four inner lights of the matrix were orange, the eight outer lights blue, and the whole covered by a thin black cloth. The illumination of the display was 4.11 cd/m^2. An observer watching through a one-way mirror recorded visual fixation times using an event recorder.

The stimulus was presented for 30 seconds followed by a 10-second intertrial period. After six presentations, the stimulus was changed to a simpler pattern (four green lights in the form of a square). For each stimulus presentation, the length of time the child kept his eyes on the stimulus after intitial fixation was noted. The least squares slope of the six initial fixation times was calculated. Larger negative values of this slope reflect diminishing attention to this repeated stimulus, and are interpreted as indicating more rapid habituation (response decrement). A second measure, recovery of attention (dishabituation), was the duration, in seconds, of the child's initial fixation on the changed stimulus of the seventh trial, minus the duration of fixation on the sixth trial.

Children were tested in a single session. The procedures were administered in the following order: 1) the Bayley mental scale, with the object–permanence test incorporated, 2) the Bayley motor scale, 3) the observation of free play, 4) the visual habituation and dishabituation tests. Examiners were not aware of a mother's treatment group assignment. Supplemented mothers did not themselves know whether they had been given the high protein Supplement or the balanced protein/calorie Complement. Of course they were aware of whether or not their diet had been supplemented.

Rationale for Choice of Measures

Cognitive competence was the outcome of central interest, and we tried to select tests that might meet three desiderata: First, the test should reflect motor and social development at the age of examination. In this study developmental stage was indicated by the Bayley mental and motor scales, and by the two Piagetian-type measures (object–permanence and sophistication of play).

Second, the test should to some degree predict later intellectual competence. A relationship to later mental competence has been found with the Bayley tests. We hoped to strengthen prediction by using a battery of tests. The tests of visual habituation and observation of play were included to expand the battery.

Lewis [1971] had suggested that habituation might be a sensitive index of early intellectual development. Lewis' series was small, and the subjects drawn from a population dissimilar to our own, but he reported correlations of $r = 0.46$ and 0.50 between measures of habituation to a visual stimulus at age one and subsequent intellectual development as measured by Stanford-Binet tests at 40 months of age. Observations of play behavior were intended to provide an analogue for studies of exploratory behavior in animals, which in them had seemed to relate to cognitive competence.

Third, we hoped to find tests that were sensitve to nutritional change. Experimental and observational studies on children malnourished in early life have pointed to a wide range of developmental deficits at age one. With regard to habituation, Lester [1975] noted that ill-grown one-year-old Guatemalan children did not respond to auditory stimulation, and therefore could not habituate, while well-grown children performed as expected. With regard to play, studies of animal behavior suggest that nutritionally deprived animals are less likely to explore in an open field, as also to maintain attention or to manipulate objects [Dobbing and Smart, 1973; Frankova, 1974; Levitsky, 1973]. These behaviors have frequently occurred in malnourished animals in the absence of specific learning deficits.

RESULTS

Somatic Measures and Treatment (Table 4.1)

One-year-old infants were compared across treatment groups on six measures of somatic development: height, weight, head circumference, arm girth, and thickness of skinfolds over the triceps and subscapular areas. All measures were adjusted for age and sex. No significant effects of treatment were found for any of the somatic measures, all of which are correlated with each other.* Conditional effects that might be anticipated from the modification of treatment effects on birthweight by length of gestation at birth, and on maternal weight gain by stage of gestation at entry to treatment, were not found. (Appendix 4.2). The

---

*Correlations ranged from $r = 0.22$ ($p < 0.01$) between triceps skinfold and length, to $r = 0.58$ ($p < 0.001$) between triceps and subscapular skinfolds. The only correlation that was not significant was between length and subscapular skinfold.

TABLE 4.1. Somatic Measures at One Year of Age by Treatment

Measure	Treatment Group			
	Supplement Mean (n)	Complement Mean (n)	Control Mean (n)	Total Mean ± SD
Weight (kg)	9.629 (202)	9.568 (207)	9.497 (217)	9.563 ± 1.267
Height (inches)	0.749 (204)	0.747 (208)	0.747 (220)	0.747 ± 0.30
Head circumference (cm)	46.08 (204)	45.97 (208)	46.03 (219)	46.03 ± 1.53
Arm girth (cm)	15.67 (203)	15.56 (205)	15.56 (218)	15.59 ± 1.53
Triceps skinfold (mm)	8.45 (204)	8.36 (203)	8.53 (217)	8.45 ± 2.38
Subscapular skinfold (mm)	7.19 (103)	6.29 (204)	6.99 (216)	7.03 ± 1.93
Age at Examination (days)	348 (205)	357*(208)	348 (220)	351 ± 48

Mean for each measure (numbers examined in parentheses) and standard deviation of total. All measures adjusted for chronologic age and sex.

*$p < 0.05$, vs other two groups combined.

infants born prematurely in the high protein Supplement group (in which fetal growth was slowed and mortality raised) were not growth retarded at age one. Infants born to mothers who entered treatment before 15 weeks gestation showed no advantage over those whose mothers entered after 15 weeks.

Psychological Measures and Treatment (Table 4.2)

The infants were compared on ten measures of psychological development: Bayley mental scale, Bayley motor scale, object-permanence test, observations of play (sophistication, latency to leave the mother, mean length of episodes, number of rectangles**, number of episodes**), and visual habituation and dishabituation. All measures were adjusted for age and sex. For seven psychological measures (Bayley motor scale, Bayley mental scale, object-permanence, latency, number of rectangles, sophistication of play, number of episodes), no significant differences were found among treatment groups.

For three measures (habituation, dishabituation, length of play episodes) significant differences were found. In each instance,

**Not shown in Table 4.2.

TABLE 4.2. Psychological Measures at One Year of Age by Treatment

Measure	Treatment group			Total mean ± SD
	Supplement mean (n)	Complement mean (n)	Control mean (n)	
Bayley mental score	98.97 (199)	98.65 (197)	99.39 (214)	99.01 ± 6.23
Bayley motor score	45.78 (201)	45.79 (203)	45.81 (216)	45.79 ± 3.47
Object permanence score	14.95 (159)	14.75 (163)	15.12 (164)	14.94 ± 3.75
Play: latency (secs)	125 (143)	129 (136)	108 (150)	120 ± 207
sophistication (median score)	4.27 (130)	4.17 (119)	4.33 (136)	4.26 ± (1.12)
Mean length of episode (secs)	87.3* (144)	59.7 (136)	71.7 (148)	73.2 ± 89.2
Habituation (slope)	−0.84** (124)	−0.57* (131)	−0.66 (135)	−0.69 ± 0.77
Dishabituation (secs)	4.6* (127)	2.2 (123)	1.3 (126)	2.7 ± 11.7

Mean for each measure (numbers examined in parentheses) and standard deviation of total. All measures adjusted for chronologic age and sex.

* p < 0.05, vs other 2 groups combined

**p < 0.01, vs other 2 groups combined

the Supplement group scores were significantly different from the other two groups combined. For all three measures the Supplement group scores were also different from the Complement group scores, although the difference for dishabituation was not statistically significant. By contrast, the Complement group scores were not significantly different from the Control group scores on any measure. As with the somatic measures, there was no evidence of depressed psychological function among infants born prematurely in the Supplement group; also the infants whose mothers entered treatment early showed no particular advantage (Appendix 4.2).

The structure of relationships among the contemporary somatic and psychological measures and birthweight is instructive. The five somatic measures, as well as six of the seven psychological measures that did not relate to treatment, are substantially intercorrelated. (Latency, the interval before the child left the mother to enter an adjacent rectangle, did not correlate with treatment, nor with the other measures.) Further, these two sets of somatic and psychological measures not only correlate with each other, but are correlated with length of gestation and birthweight; these variables also do not relate significantly to treatment. Appendices 4.3 and 4.4 show that these outcomes, more particularly the somatic measures, relate also to maternal predictors of birthweight (ponderal index at conception, arm girth, education and welfare status, previous low birthweight deliveries) and to other indices of fetal growth at birth (placental weight, newborn infant length, and head circumference) as well as to chronologic age at testing. We designate the six psychological measures that correlate with somatic measures as "growth related."

In striking contrast, the three psychological measures that at age one did relate to treatment show virtually no significant associations either with the 11 growth-related measures, or with birthweight, or with predictors of birthweight, or even with age at testing. Among these three measures, habituation and dishabituation are structurally related and correlated with each other. Neither of the two shows an association with the third measure, namely, length of play episodes. We designate these three psychological measures that relate only to Supplement as "protein related."

Control of Confounding (Appendix 4.5)

In further analyses, we aimed to eliminate confounding, which might lead us spuriously to infer that treatment produced the protein-related outcomes, and suppression, which might prevent us from detecting treatment effects [Susser, 1973]. Each outcome variable was subjected to several hierarchal multiple regression analyses, with differing sets of independent variables entered into the equation in a predetermined way. One sequence of independent variables was similar to that used in the previous chapters for analyzing maternal weight gain and birthweight. In this sequence, we controlled for those variables used initially to stratify the sample population, and also for maternal smoking. Another sequence controlled for variables most strongly associated with psychological development. We also entered a large number of interaction terms (for treatment and other independent variables) into the equations. None of these statistical procedures modify in any but trivial ways the relationship between treatment and outcome set out above. They therefore set at rest some reasonable objections to making strong inferences from the findings.

Some Regression Analyses (Appendix 4.5)

Bayley Mental Score (Appendix 4.5a) – Several significant relationships with this score persisted in a multiple regression analysis which controlled for several potentially confounding factors. The score had negative relationships with the number of past low birthweight deliveries and with later registration for prenatal care; and positive ones with duration of gestation, birthweight, and caloric intake during the study. After controlling for length of gestation, a negative relationship with treatment by Complement became significant; this is of questionable importance, since the Complement group had longer duration of gestation.

Bayley Motor Score (Appendix 4.5b) – As with the Bayley mental score, the motor score had negative relationships with history of past low birthweight, and with later registration for prenatal care, and positive relationships with duration of gestation and birthweight. There were no significant relationships with treatment.

Habituation (Appendix 4.5c) – The *only* significant relationship of this measure was with Supplement ($F = 8.13$, $P < 0.001$).

The relationship with protein intake was not significant.

Dishabituation (Appendix 4.5d) — This measure too was significantly related to Supplement ($F = 5.16$, $P < 0.05$). The simple relationship of protein intake and dishabituation was not significant. An obscure and complicated relationship of dishabituation with protein intake seems to exist, however. After calorie intake was controlled in the regression equation, a significant negative relationship with protein intake appeared. We are unable to interpret this finding.

Duration of episodes of play (Appendix 4.5e) — The *only* significant relationship of this measure was with Supplement treatment vs all others ($F=6.17$, $0.01<P<0.05$).

Treatment, Premature Birth, and Outcome

In view of the implied adverse outcome of high-protein prenatal supplementation on premature births, special interest attaches itself to the effect of treatment on outcome among this group at one year of age. First, there were no detectable adverse outcomes among them. When premature infants were taken separately (Appendix 4.2), only one of the three protein-related outcomes (dishabituation) showed a treatment effect in the same direction as in the total group. The correlations with treatment of the other two protein-related outcomes, habituation and length of play episodes, were near zero. Although the numbers of prematures are small, these results give no suggestion of any residual toxic effect.

DISCUSSION

Among infants of mothers selected for a test of prenatal nutritional intervention, results for outcome measures around one year of age fell into two distinct classes, one unrelated and the other strongly related to treatment.

In one class, six intercorrelated psychological outcome measures could be described as *growth related.* That is, these psychological measures correlated with somatic measures at one year of age, and both sets correlated with indices of growth at birth. Since prenatal nutritional treatment had had no detectable favorable effect on birthweight, it is no surprise that it had no detectable effect on these measures of outcome.

In a second contrasting class, three psychological measures of outcome could be described as *protein related*. These measures correlate weakly or not at all with the growth-related measures and with birthweight, but they relate significantly to high protein treatment. Clearly, an effect of prenatal nutritional treatment on the protein-related outcomes must be direct and not mediated through fetal growth. We know of nothing in the literature which could have led us to hypothesize so sharp a separation of protein-related and growth-related outcomes.

Among the three protein-related outcomes, there is a further dissociation of the visual habituation measures from the play measure. Habituation and dishabituation are correlated with each other in a manner expected for two facets of the same phenomenon. Length of play episodes is not correlated with either of the habituation measures, and can be regarded as independently related to the high-protein treatment.

One must ask if the positive results of psychological outcomes at one year of age have been subjected to sufficiently rigorous statistical testing. Although the experimental design meets the conventions for the formal testing of specified hypotheses, some of the positive results would not retain significance in the face of more stringent criteria for testing multiple outcomes. The result is reinforced, however, by the patterned and coherent structure of growth-related and protein-related measures. Although one must expect a proportion of significant results merely from the play of chance, the expectation that chance will produce a coherent set of positive and negative results to the advantage of the main experimental group is considerably small.

One may yet ask whether the failure to demonstrate treatment effects in the growth-related variables is not owed to a lack of power to detect positive results that are present. Statistical power was not determined at the outset. There was no way of predicting the size of effect of prenatal supplementation on the one year psychological measures, and sample size was derived from the test of effect on birthweight. Analysis on completion of the study shows that for each outcome measure, the power to detect a difference of 20% of a standard deviation in the means of the treated and control groups ranges from 35% to 50%, depending on sample size. The power to detect an effect of this size is no bigger for the protein-related measures than for the growth-related measures. Moreover, the results on tests which showed no significant effect of treatment have no consistent direction, and do not suggest that effects of small size have been missed.

The dissociation of growth- and protein-related outcomes opens up new areas of speculation. Here we discuss a few of the questions.

The Meaning of the Protein-Related Measures

Lewis [1971] writes of visual habituation tests that "those infants and young children who show response decrement are those subjects with more efficient central nervous system function." To support this assertion, Lewis cites findings that response decrement is more rapid at later ages, with higher socioeconomic status, with more intensive mother-infant interaction, and in children with superior performance in problem-solving tests. In one series of children, habituation at 13 months of age correlated with the Stanford-Binet IQ at four years of age.

Our finding therefore suggests superiority of mental function in the children exposed prenatally to the high protein Supplement. A study from Guatemala may point in the same direction. Lester [1975] found that a group of 20 well-grown one-year-old infants, after orienting in response to an auditory stimulus, became habituated to its repetition, and then responded afresh to a changed stimulus. A group of 20 ill-grown infants of comparable family background showed no response at all to the auditory stimulus. Responses were inferred from cardiac rate as well as from observed behavior. In this study, however, nutritional state was indirectly inferred from height and weight and thus the differences in response are growth-related, although the difference in growth may have been incidental. Further, the stimulus is not the same as in our study, and the recorded responses occurred, one must assume, at one extreme of the range of possible responses, since in the ill-grown children response curves were flat. In the absence of responses, response decrement cannot be considered as having been measured among them.

A recently published observation from a study in Bogotá [Vuori et al, 1979] may also be relevant. Visual habituation in 15-day-old infants was more rapid in prenatally supplemented group than in randomly-assigned controls. The measure did not correlate with birthweight (which showed some response to supplementation) nor with other measures of observed behavior. This result, compatible with ours, is incompatible with Lewis' view that the mental schemata and memory functions for the appreciation of a novel stimulus do not develop before three months of age.

Another unpublished study of squirrel monkeys found that visual habituation in two- and three-year-old monkeys varied with their exposure to different nutritional and social conditions from two through nine weeks of age [Boelkins and Hegsted, 1978]. Smaller differences were produced by experimental variation of nutritional conditions than of social conditions, however. In younger monkeys, at one year of age, habituation did not relate to nutrition. Dishabituation did not relate to nutrition at any age.

These isolated observations on habituation gain new significance when linked to the strong inference that can be made from the present randomized controlled trial of nutritional supplementation. Yet the variability in the conditions of testing and in the outcomes cannot all be accomodated by extant theories, even if these were in accord and not competing.

There is disagreement about the meaning of the length of play episodes. Kagan [1971] regards these as a measure of "conceptual tempo" and of "reflexivity-impulsivity." He found longer play episodes in children (especially girls) of higher socio economic status. Longer play episodes, Pederson and Wender [1968] found in two and a half-year-old boys, also related to higher performance scores on the Wechsler Intelligence Scale for Children at six years of age. To the contrary, Lewis [1971] reported shorter episodes of play with higher socio economic status, and cited a study [Hutt, 1968] in which longer episodes were associated with brain damage.

We find no grounds for choosing between these opposing sets of results. The stalemate need not preclude our choosing between interpretations. Kagan's views on play episodes combined with Lewis' views on habituation permit consistency in the interpretation of our results. Both longer play episodes and rapid habituation would be seen as favorable outcomes. Our large series, specifically generated to test an hypothesis, lends credibility to this interpretation of the effect of high protein supplementation.

Protein Levels and Protein-Related Measures

In the present study, the high protein Supplement produced a substantial increment in prenatal protein intake among women who on an average were already on an adequate protein diet. The effect seems most likely to be specific to protein, or to a protein constituent. Any effect of nonprotein constituents should have been apparent with Complement but the balanced protein-calorie treatment had no influence on either habituation measures nor on length of play episodes. Relative to Supplement, Complement supplied substantially less protein. It supplied somewhat fewer calories in total, and similar amounts of nonprotein.

These effects can perhaps best be seen as the result of a high booster dose of protein over and above "normal" nutritional needs. The concept of a booster follows by elimination from the absence either of a linear response to dose or of a conditional response to maternal nutritional state. No response to dose across treatment groups was evident (although possibly the extra protein in Complement was too little for a test of linearity). There is also no suggestion of a response conditional on nutritional status; the effects were unrelated to the mother's prepregnant weight or to weight gain during pregnancy.

The apparent independence of the Supplement treatment effects from size at birth opens the question of timing and critical periods. Maternal nutrition has had detectable effects on fetal growth predominantly in the third trimester of pregnancy [Smith, 1947; Bergner and Susser, 1970; Stein and Susser, 1975]. Thus, disassociation of growth- and protein-related measures might follow from protein effects produced early in pregnancy. This hypothesis can be put aside. Entry into treatment early in pregnancy did not differentiate the mothers whose infants showed the protein effects from those who did not.

The independence of the treatment effects from nutritional state and dose of Supplement, as well as timing, provokes the thought that the stimulus resides in change itself, that is, in the abrupt alteration of an accustomed protein balance. (When faced with the adverse effect of the high protein Supplement on length of gestation and fetal growth, we likewise considered the possibility that abrupt dietary change had provoked a failure of adaptation). The estimated average daily protein intake in the Supplement group (102 gm) was 35% greater than in the Control group (79 gm); by contrast, in the Complement group protein intake (83 gm) was only 5% greater. In Bogotá, in the supplemented group in which an effect was found in the newborn, estimated daily protein intake was boosted by 57%, from 35 gm to 55 gm.

The results for habituation in the newborn in the Bogotá study, and in squirrel monkeys exposed to early malnutrition in the Boelkins and Hegsted study, may or may not be relevant to our results. In contrast to our study, supplementation in Bogotá provided an increment to the diet of women who were undernourished by almost any standard. In the squirrel monkey study, the factorial design is said not to have discriminated between the effects of calorie deprivation associated with the two different levels of protein deprivation, whether the proportion of total calories supplied by protein was 12%, or 3.5 to 5%. Thus among infants in Bogotá the result is owed to the action of supplements in women at a much poorer level of nutrition than in the New York population, and in the squirrel monkey study the level of calorie intake, given protein deprivation, seems not to be germane to the outcome. The explanation for these discrepancies is obscure, and they may be resolved in the future.

One-Year Outcome and Adverse Outcome at Birth

The possible persistence of adverse effects in the high protein Supplement treatment group is a matter of high theoretical and practical concern. Intrauterine growth retardation, shortened gestation, and excess newborn death were limited to those born prematurely. In terms of growth-related measures, prematures in the Supplement group show no residua in comparison with either Complement and Control groups or with the mature Supplement group. In terms of protein-related measures also, they show no residua in comparison with Complement and Control groups.

On two of the three protein-related measures, however, the entire treatment effect resided among mature births. The absence of positive response among the prematures also seems unlikely to be the result of a residual adverse effect, since there are no differences from the Complement and

Control groups born at term. A partial explanation may be that the less mature infants may not yet have been ready to respond to habituation [Lewis, 1971]. Boelkins and Hegsted [1978], for example, did not find the nutrition-related habituation responses in one-year-old monkeys that they found in two- and three-year-old monkeys.

CONCLUSION

The effects of the high protein prenatal Supplement on measures of habituation and play appear not to be conditional on initial nutritional state, and they do not conform with a linear dose-response mode. We conclude that the Supplement produced two independent treatment effects on psychological performance at one year of age: one on habituation/dishabituation, the other on duration of play episodes. The biological significance of these effects we take to be favorable. Further, no appreciable residua of the adverse effects of the high protein Supplement detected at birth are detectable at age one.

SUMMARY

In a randomized controlled trial of prenatal nutritional supplementation, the offspring were assessed at around one year of age. One treatment group was given a high protein beverage (Supplement), a second was given a beverage with balanced protein and calories (Complement), and a third was given routine clinic vitamin and mineral supplements in the form of tablets (Control). Outcome is reported with respect to six somatic measures (weight, height, head circumference, arm-girth, triceps skinfold, subscapular skinfold) and ten psychological measures (Bayley mental scale, Bayley motor scale, a test of object-permanence, observations of free play yielding five measures, a test of visual habituation and one of dishabituation). No significant effects of treatment were found on any of the somatic measures, nor on seven of the psychological measures. Significant effects of the high protein Supplement were found on three psychological measures: visual habituation, visual dishabituation, and the mean length of free play episodes.

Six of the seven psychological measures that did not show treatment effects were correlated with each other, and with the somatic measures at one year. They were also correlated with duration of gestation, birthweight, and other somatic measures at birth. These psychological and somatic measures together are termed "growth-related" outcomes. By contrast, the three measures showing significant effects of high protein Supplement correlated neither with other one-year outcome measures nor with perinatal outcome measures. They are termed "protein-related" outcomes. Two of these, visual habituation and visual dishabituation, were correlated with each other; the third (length of play episodes) was not correlated with either of the other two. The three protein-related outcomes were not affected by the balanced protein/calorie Complement.

The findings suggest that prenatal high protein supplementation influences a set of psychological measures that are unrelated to physical growth, but does not influence another set of somatic and psychological measures that are related to growth. The direction of effects of the high protein Supplement is assumed to be favorable. The group of prematurely born offspring among whom adverse prenatal and perinatal protein effects occurred exhibited no residual adverse effects at one year of age.

Chapter V

Prenatal Nutritional, Quasi, and Natural Experiments in the Past Decade: An Overview*

INTRODUCTION

In the review of the literature on the effects of prenatal nutrition on fetal growth with which we initiated the current study [Bergner and Susser, 1970], we found that most of our knowledge derived from observational studies. Controlled trials of nutritional supplementation, we concluded, would be timely. Now, in a review of work in the past decade, we can draw new knowledge from a number of controlled trials or quasi-experimental** studies of prenatal supplementation. The new generation of studies was built on the shortcomings of past studies to attain rigor of design and relied on the speed and flexibility of computers to pursue complex analyses. Though gains in substantive knowledge may seem modest, the pattern of results begins to show some consistency.

Table 5.1 lists ten studies known to us, while Appendix 5.1 gives details of six. Five are trials of nutritional supplementation. Aside from our New York study, two have been fairly fully described in the literature; they were carried out in

---

*A main part of the material in this chapter is adapted from Stein, Susser, and Rush, J Repro Med 21:287–299, 1978.
**We use the term quasi-experimental to classify studies that lie in the grey area between experimental and observational studies. Typical experimental studies test the effects of specified *interventions* in a *predesignated* group by comparison with other *predesignated* groups similar in all respects but the intervention. Typical observational studies test effects of specified *exposures* (known or assumed) in groups *not predesignated*. Quasi-experimental studies may have specific interventions, but either an experimental or a comparison group or both are not predesignated. The term natural experiment is here used to describe observational studies of the effects of sharp, well-defined but unplanned change in which the time-sequence of cause and effect is clear and the exposed and unexposed comparison groups can be readily identified.

Table 5.1. Ten Recent or Ongoing Studies

Site	Investigators
New York	Rush, Stein, Susser
Bogotá	Mora, Herrera
Guatemala	Habicht, Yarbrough, Lechtig, Klein
Montreal	Higgins, Rush
Netherlands	Stein, Susser, Saenger, Marolla
Taiwan	Blackwell, Blackwell, Herriot, Hsueh, Aitchison (previously, Chow)
Bombay	Merchant, Sheth
Cardiff	Elwood et al
Aberdeen	Campbell, MacGillivray, Johnstone
Birmingham	Wharton

Bogotá, Colombia [Mora et al, 1979] and Guatemala [Habicht et al, 1974]. We will also discuss an intervention study carried out in Montreal,* uncontrolled in execution but controlled in the analysis, and an extended study of the Dutch famine of 1944–45 [Stein et al, 1975]. The Dutch study can be described as a natural experiment; that is, a sharp, time-limited change in circumstances in a well-demarcated area conferred on this observational study some advantages of experimental studies. In particular, the classification of exposed and unexposed groups was secure, the degree and timing of exposure were measurable, and above all, the time sequence of hypothesized cause and effect was unambiguous. The Montreal and Dutch studies, as well as the New York study, are our own and necessarily benefit in exposition from that circumstance. Some studies in which the results are as yet scanty or unavailable are lightly covered or merely tabulated. The rest are summarized in Appendix 5.1.

At delivery birthweight is the main outcome considered. Information on birthweight is far more comprehensive and reliable than that on other fetal dimensions, such as head size, length, and ponderal index. At later ages, we shall also consider psychological outcomes, although results for this domain are as yet limited.

---

*This study is based on the work of Mrs. Agnes Higgins. It has been evaluated by David Rush and submitted for publication.

The New York Study

In New York we were concerned with the high rate of low birthweight infants born to poor black women who were presumed to be poorly nourished. Attributes of low income black women who were at especially high risk of bearing low birthweight infants were first identified in preliminary studies [Rush, Davis, Susser, 1972]. A target population was selected on the basis of these attributes.

In short, this randomized, partially double-blind controlled trial of prenatal supplementation carried out among poor women in a typical inner city in the United States has yielded paradoxical results. The data indicate that the women used the beverage appropriately. The beverages had no significant effect on birthweight. Women on the balanced protein-calorie Complement had an advantage in birthweight of 41 gm over controls and fewer low birthweight infants. Those women on high protein Supplement had a disadvantage in birthweight of 42 gm; they had high rates of very premature delivery and neonatal death and, among prematures, retarded growth. Conditional effects were present in both directions: Women with previously low birthweight infants responded adversely to the high protein Supplement; women who were heavy smokers responded favorably to both Supplement and Complement. Among the majority who gave birth *at term,* the birthweights of the supplemented groups were in the expected direction, but the difference between the extreme groups was only 24 gm, well below the difference anticipated in the study. Similarly, around one year of age the infants of supplemented mothers showed no advantages in either physical growth or in a battery of psychological measures that were highly correlated with growth and with each other. Yet the infants of mothers on the high protein Supplement showed effects on psychological measures quite unrelated to measurable growth.

Given that the nutritional supplements were used — and the evidence is strong that they were — we must conclude from the New York study that, in United States populations at high risk of low birthweight, maternal diet during pregnancy has modest effects on birthweight except in heavy smokers.

Maternal starvation in the latter part of pregnancy lowers birthweight, but only when dietary intake falls below a threshold. It turned out that the diets of the New York women, contrary to prevailing opinion, were deficient in calories but not in protein. At the same time, the study suggests that a pathway exists between protein supplementation and psychological function that is independent of gross somatic development. This response may represent a booster effect, the converse of a limiting threshold.

The Montreal Study [Rush et al, 1976]

In a large Montreal hospital prenatal clinic serving a low-income population it was the practice to refer unselected women to the nutrition service supplied by the Montreal Diet Dispensary; both dietary advice and supplements could be given.* The hospital maintained careful, computerized records for all deliveries, including birthweight and other data. Records of mothers who were not referred to the service provided retrospectively selected controls. These comparison mothers were matched to those using the nutrition service on a number of characteristics: year of delivery, religion, gravidity, prepregnant weight, and trimester of entering prenatal care.

Although the nutritional intervention in this case was not a controlled trial, the quasi-experimental design yielded useful findings for our purposes. The study women were public patients, and therefore presumed to be poor. Their diets were probably inadequate, although these women, like those in the New York study, were not overtly malnourished. The type of intervention was sometimes limited to advice, but about three-quarters were given foodstuffs. Smoking was recorded only for subjects, and then, only late in the study.

Among the offspring of women referred to the Diet Dispensary, mean birthweight was about 40 gm greater than in the comparison group (Table 5.2). In this large sample the difference was statistically significant ($p < 0.05$). The frequency of low birthweight was

---

*In the first phase of this program the women referred to the Montreal Diet Dispensary were those who registered on certain days of the week. Later, every other woman who registered at the prenatal clinic was referred to the Diet Dispensary.

Table 5.2. Montreal Study

	Referred to Diet Dispensary	Matched controls	p value
All (1213 pairs)	3291 ± 508	3251 ± 510	<0.05
Primiparae* (478 pairs)	3218 ± 482	3157 ± 502	<0.05
Lighter weight women < 140 lbs preconception (998 pairs)	3248 ± 482	3195 ± 481	<0.02
Lighter weight primiparae (439 pairs)	3203 ± 481	3130	<0.02

Mean birthweight in grams (±SD) among women referred to Diet Dispensary and matched controls.

*47 pairs included a woman with history of low birthweight delivery. When excluded, the supplement/control difference remained identical (61 gm).

5.7% among those referred, as compared with 6.8% in the controls. This advantage is not statistically significant. The effect on birthweight of referral to dietary treatment was again conditional. Thus, as compared to their matched controls, primiparae had a 61 gm advantage, and women who weighed less than 140 lbs at conception had a 53 gm advantage. Women who were both primiparae and weighed less than 140 lbs at conception had a 73 gm advantage. In the New York study only women who weighed under 140 lbs were recruited, but light women on supplements who weighed under 110 lbs at conception also had infants with more favorable birthweight than did lightweight controls, although the differences were not statistically significant.

Another result of the Montreal study requires serious consideration despite lack of statistical significance. For women who had previous low birthweight infants, referral to the Diet Dispensary was associated with *lower* birthweights than untreated controls with the same history, just as in those women assigned to the high-protein Supplement in the New York study. In Montreal, also, these women had depressed weight gain during pregnancy as well as shortened duration of gestation compared to controls with the same history.

The results of the Montreal study are consistent with those of the New York study. From these results we conclude that prenatal supplementation can be expected to produce a modest increment in birthweight among women who are underweight and who are by inference underfed. The results also warn that previously unsuspected harm could follow from nutritional treatment. In the New York study a toxic contaminant in the beverage is a highly unlikely explanation of the adverse effect, which is difficult to rule out entirely. The apparent adverse effect among Montreal women who had previously had low birthweight infants, and who were given supplements of regular foodstuffs only, goes some way towards ruling it out.

It remains for us to examine the effect of dietary supplementation in chronically malnourished populations and in further studies of acute maternal starvation. From a worldwide perspective, the South American studies to be described next are therefore of great significance.

The Bogotá Study [Mora et al, 1979]

The Bogotá study is a randomized controlled trial of both prenatal and postnatal intervention. Both nutritional and psychological treaments were tested, although neither of them could be given blind. Families living in a poor urban environment were randomly selected. They and families clustered around them were given supplements to their regular diet (considered deficient in calories and protein) of about 1,600 calories and 25.5 gm of protein daily. A control series was identified in the same manner before the supplements were given, and these families, like those supplemented, were observed through and after pregnancy. For a family to be eligible for the trial, "malnutrition" had to be present in at least 50% of the children under 5 years of age (primigravidae were presumably not enrolled).

Women were introduced to the nutrional treatment in two phases—at the sixth month of pregnancy, and six months after birth of the child. Both food supplementation schedules continued up to three years of age. Psychosocial stimulation introduced at birth. These treatments were combined in a factorial design to generate six treatment groups in all. For the test of the effects of prenatal supplementation alone, however, these could be reduced to two groups. The prenatal supplements, which consisted of milk, cooking oil, and enriched bread, were instituted in the sixth month of pregnancy.

In the Bogotá study, among supplemented mothers, infant birthweight was 60 gm higher, and the proportion of low birthweight infants was reduced (Table 5.3). The result was significant on a one-tailed test. On a two-tailed test, which the adverse New York result would seem to demand, neither of the results was significant at $p < 0.05$. That is not surprising because the trial was not designed to detect so small an increment. Evidence that the women themselves did share in the extra food was provided by twice-repeated dietary recalls. The mean increment to the diet, as indicated by the mean of two 24-hour dietary histories, was 136 calories and 20 gm of protein. Thin women, but not heavy women, had a significant increment in calorie intake, although both groups increased their protein intake. In parallel, infants of thin women were 181gm heavier than those of controls; infants of heavy women were only 22 gm heavier. As in the New York high protein Supplement group, the average weight gain during pregnancy was higher among the supplemented. Results were not analyzed in terms of duration of treatment. Perinatal mortality was halved in the supplemented group, although numbers were too small for statistical significance.

TABLE 5.3. Bogotá Study

Length of gestation	Supplemented	Unsupplemented	Difference in gm
Boys			
Full term	3,061 ± 376 (95)	2,947 ± 332 (76)	+114
Preterm	2,874 (12)	2,901 (20)	− 27
All	3,040 ± 414 (107)	2,939 ± 414 (96)	+101
Girls			
Full term	2,935 ± 316 (82)	2,935 ± 30 (89)	0
Preterm	2,749 (19)	2,679 (20)	+ 70
All	2,900 ± 339 (101)	2,888 ± 394 (109)	+ 12
Both sexes			
Full term	3,003 ± 354 (177)	2,940 ± 318 (165)	+ 63
Preterm	2,797 (31)	2,790 (40)	+ 7
All	2,972 ± 385 (208)	2,912 ± 404 (205)	+ 60

Mean birthweight in gm (±SD) for supplemented and unsupplemented maternities by sex. Numbers of births in parentheses.

An intriguing finding of the Bogotá study was that the gain in birthweight for the supplemented families was confined entirely to male births. Moreover, during the third trimester when fetal growth contributes appreciably to maternal weight gain, mothers who bore sons gained more weight and also ate slightly more than those who bore daughters. Among unsupplemented mothers such differences according to the sex of the infants were not found.

An adverse result comparable to that of the New York study was not evident in the Bogotá study. Certainly, the proportion of low birthweight infants was not increased. Among premature deliveries, although supplemented preterm boys weighed 27 gm less than unsupplemented ones, supplemented preterm girls were 70 gm heavier than the unsupplemented ones. Data on women in Bogotá who had previously had low birthweight offspring have not been reported. The effect of smoking, too, has not been reported on, but smoking is infrequent among these women.

Detailed monitoring of the mothers' dietary intake in this study was complicated by a design that relied on family supplementation to achieve adequate diet for all members. No doubt, also, there will be further and more detailed analysis of weight gain patterns, with control of the duration of treatment and the stage of gestation at entry into treatment. Meanwhile, this controlled trial among malnourished families supports the view that additional food given in the third trimester can raise birthweight to some degree. The gain was modest, and for the given magnitude of effect, the numbers were at the lower margin of sufficiency for achieving statistical significance.

The only psychological outcome so far reported is an effect of supplementation on visual habituation in the postnatal period. As in the New York study among infants around one year of age, the supplemented infants habituated more rapidly than controls (Vuori et al, 1979).

The Guatemala Study [Habicht et al, 1974]

Mothers and children living in each of four small villages in Guatemala were encouraged to come daily to a supplementation center, where they were invited to partake ad lib of a liquid diet supplement. In two villages the supplement was fortified with protein in addition to calories, vitamins and minerals; in the others it was not. The amount taken by each person was noted at each visit.

The daily diet of the villagers consisted of about 1,500 calories, including some 40 gm of protein. This protein intake was considerably lower than among unsupplemented New York women and slightly higher than among those in Bogotá. The usual proportion of infants born at weights less than 2,500 gm was given by the investigators as 20%, somewhat less than the rate expected among the high-risk women selected for the New York study. In this study, as in New York, there was detailed documentation of dietary supplementation, of somatic measures of mothers and infants, and of developmental measures of infants, although systematic placental studies were lacking. The Guatemala study also provided for every woman a measure of beverage ingestion from direct observation, which the New York and Bogotá studies could not.

Infants were weighed as soon as possible after a birth was reported, usually on the first day. Birthweights and supplementation were analyzed for 405, or 62%, of the 648 known births. In the last three years of the study, this rate rose to 92%. Under the circumstances, a considerable loss of information was probably inevitable. Because of potential bias among these losses, the reports presented so far are vulnerable to confounding, since losses are more likely to have occurred among unexpectedly premature births, stillbirths, and early neonatal deaths, which in undeveloped societies often go unreported. The reported data do not speak to the point of possible adverse effects of high protein supplementation; for this we must await a further analysis of total births, including the premature births and perinatal losses.

The initial experiment was designed to contrast the effects of protein supplements with those of protein-free supplements across villages. Comparisons of protein- and nonprotein-supplemented villages, however, did not reveal the expected advantages of the protein supplement. On the supposition that effects of supplementation might be masked because both forms were effective, the investigators abandoned the preset experimental comparison in favor of post hoc comparisons between individual women according to their measured caloric supplementation, irrespective of the form or protein content of the beverage. In this quasi-experimental analysis, birthweight was shown to relate to the quantity of supplemental calories consumed during pregnancy. Differences seemed to be entirely attributable to total calories in the diet and not to the amount of protein. The phase of pregnancy at which the calories were ingested, it was also reported, did not affect birthweight.

A regression analysis suggests that a total ingestion of 20,000 extra calories over the 280 days of pregnancy (or about 70 calories per day) resulted in a gain of 56 gm in birthweight (the various reports of the study differ somewhat on this estimate; we have chosen what appears to be the most recent). The amounts of caloric supplementation corresponding to difference in birthweight are not translatable from this analysis into daily average intake, which would permit comparison with the New York and Bogotá studies. Total ingestion is reported, but duration of treatment during pregnancy, which is needed in order to make such estimates, is not. Table 5.4 gives estimated data for 288 selected livebirths from the total of 648.

These analyses of the Guatemala trial lose the advantages of inference that inhere in the original controlled experimental design because the predetermined assignments of supplement were made among villages and not among individual women. In each village the mothers themselves chose whether to visit

TABLE 5.4. Guatemala Study

	Supplemental calories	
	$<20,000$	$\geq 20,000$
Birthweight	2,996 ± 450	3,220 ± 500
No.	171	117
% > 3,500 gm	9.9	20.9
% 2,500–3,500 gm	80.1	75.6
% < 2,500 gm	9.9	3.5

Mean birthweight in gm (±SD), and percent distribution in 3 birthweight categories, according to amount of supplemental calories ingested in 288 full term livebirths.

the distribution centers, and if they did visit, they themselves chose the quantity of beverage they would imbibe. Hence, it could be that those women who chose to take more supplement did so because their own characteristics or those of the fetuses stimulated the appetite; determinants of appetite could also be determinants of birthweight. As noted earlier Thomson [1959], who reported an association between caloric intake and birthweight in a careful observational study in Aberdeen, considered that the association could be fully accounted for by maternal size. Although Thomson's result is open to more than one interpretation [Bergner and Susser, 1970; Stein and Susser, 1975], he argued that during pregnancy women "eat to appetite." Even in the Bogotá study it could be argued that the distinctive response in maternal weight gain and birthweight of male offspring is an expression of self-selection, in that a woman's appetite and intake may also heed the demands of the fetus.

The Guatemala investigators thus faced the classic problem in nonexperimental studies of potential confounding by the self-selection of volunteers. They were rightly concerned about whether their results could be taken to prove a causal relation between nutritional supplements and birthweight. Their analysis does put to rest a number of objections. The investigators examined the attributes of village women who did or did not choose to come to the center and who differed in the amount of supplement they drank. Maternal height and weight, morbidity, age, parity, birth interval, and home diet were considered. The researchers state that none of these factors could account for the relations between caloric ingestion and birthweight. Nor could these relations be explained by differing degrees of cooperativeness among village women, for cooperativeness was likely to influence the volume of beverage consumed, rather than the amount of calories. Calorie intake depended not only on volume but also on the nature of the supplement; the high protein supplement was three times more concentrated than the other. Also, among women observed over successive pregnancies, the infant of a later pregnancy was heavier if the mother had taken more of the supplement drink during the later pregnancy and to the degree expected from the increment in the supplement. That the intrinsic growth potential of the fetus accounted for the increased intake was unlikely, for mothers bearing boys (of heavier birthweight than girls) consumed no more than did mothers of girls.

Thus, although the Guatemala study is not a controlled trial with treatment groups designated beforehand, it supports the concept that when there is chronic malnutrition, birthweight can be raised by a sufficient caloric supplementation used throughout pregnancy. The gain in birthweight depended on the amount taken (28 gm per 10,000 total additional calories throughout pregnancy), an effect not dissimilar from that reported in the Bogotá study. The Montreal study obtained results in the same range; so, too, did the New York study, although those results were not statistically significant.

The relatively small effect on birthweight in both Guatemala and Bogotá was probably sufficient to make a difference to perinatal loss in these populations, provided the birthweight increment could be applied to the association between birthweight and perinatal mortality. Analyses of the Guatemala data indicate a nonsignificant but nonetheless convincing association of supplementation with reduced infant mortality. This reduction cannot be attributed solely to prenatal supplementation, since both infants and mothers were supplemented postnatally, and in addition, the effect of improved medical care cannot be separated from that of nutritional supplements.

The results of the Guatemala study on the effect of nutritional supplement on psychological outcome offer possible support for the hypothesis that in a malnourished human population, prenatal as well as postnatal nutrition can influence mental competence. Children were tested at 36, 48 and 60 months of age. The initial sample included 1,083 children: 671 were born during the four years of recruitment, and 412 were already born but under three years of age at the outset of the study. The actual numbers tested are not given. At each examination, on the composite measure of an array of cognitive tests as well as on several individual tests, children who were supplemented at a high average level from conception up to the time of testing scored significantly better than those who used little or no supplement. Socioeconomic status did not account for the results, and they state also that even within families, levels of supplementation related to the cognitive performance of sibs.

These results reflect prenatal and postnatal supplementation combined. The authors state that regression analyses "pinpoint the periods of gestation and of birth to 24 months as the most important in determining later mental development" [Klein et al, 1977]. From the data as reported, however, prenatal supplementation cannot be separated from postnatal supplementation either for mother or for children. With so complex an issue, the conclusion that prenatal supplementation contributed to the result cannot be taken as secure without close scrutiny of data and analyses.

The Taiwan Study [Herriot, Hsueh, and Aitchison, 1978]

The full report of the Taiwan study, which was the first of those discussed to be undertaken, is not yet in print: Publication has unfortunately been delayed by the premature death of its initiator, Bacon Chow [Blackwell et al, 1973]. An area in which nutrition was marginal and protein intake low was selected. Average daily calorie intake was estimated at 1,600 to 2,000 calories. Women with at least one male child were enrolled at the end of one pregnancy and randomly assigned to two treatment groups. In the succeeding pregnancy, a supplemented group (A) was given 40 gm of protein and 800 calories daily throughout gestation. An unsupplemented group (B) was given minerals and vitamins, and less than 40 calories per day. Procedure was double-blind. Between 125 and 128 women in each group were followed through the second test pregnancy and had their infants weighed within 24 hours of birth. After about two years of field work, a third nonintervention control group was added.

The use of the supplement was closely monitored, and the women took it under observation. About three quarters of the women took more than 50% of the supplement. This compliant group was supplemented on average by 30 gm of protein and 600 calories daily. Diet was checked in each trimester of pregnancy by a living-in nurse. These estimates of intake were extremely low: $1,133 \pm 330$ calories in Group A, $1,202 \pm 352$ calories in Group B. There was also an unexplained deficiency in the nitrogen excretion of the protein/calorie supplemented group (established on the basis of 24-hour urine specimens, taken on two occasions). Maternal weight during gestation and at term in the second test pregnancy was almost identical in the two treatment groups.

Birthweight at delivery was analyzed only for those women who used 50% or more of the supplements [Herriott, Hsueh, and Aitchison, 1978] (Table 5.5). The mean birthweight of the 81 infants of the protein/calorie supplemented women (Group A) was 94 gm higher than that of the 88 infants of control women (Group B). This advantage should perhaps be offset, however, by a 43 gm advantage in birthweight of the supplemented Group A women in the first observed pregnancy, *before* supplementation, which occurred despite randomization. Thus, a 51 gm advantage in birthweight could be ascribed to nutritional supplements. Supplemented male infants showed an advantage of 86 gm in the second test pregnancy, females of 113 gm. When the distributions of birthweights in the first observed pregnancy are offset, however, the advantage is reversed: male infants have an advantage of 79 gm, females of 39 gm.

None of these results is statistically significant. The direction of the results is as expected, the magnitude of the possible there is no sign of an adverse effect. Small numbers perhaps account for the failure to reject the null hypothesis. Yet any conclusion must be vitiated to some degree by the selectivity introduced into the experiment by the analysis. To compare results only for the women who used a sufficiency of the supplements is to allow self-selection for supplement use to determine the composition of the two treatment groups, and thus to undo the neutrality of the random assignment. No data are given that would shed light on this potential source of confounding.

At eight months of age, the children were given the Bayley tests of neuromotor behavior. Analysis was again confined to 104 offspring of mothers who took 50% or more of the prescribed supplement. Twenty-two of the 244 items were selected as exhibiting sufficient variation for analysis. One of the 22 items (bringing two objects together in midline) showed a statistically significant advantage in favor of the supplemented infants, which is about the chance expectation. Two other items leaned in the same direction ("raises self to sitting position," and "stirs with spoon in imitation"). Very little can be concluded from these results.

TABLE 5.5. Taiwan Study: Mean Birthweight in Grams (±SD)

	Group (Supplement)		Difference (gm) A–B	Untreated controls
	(A)** High protein (40 gm/d) & calorie (800 Kcal/d) supplement	(B)** Low calorie (80 Kcal/d) supplement		
Males:				
First (untreated) pregnancy				
Number	62	63	7	Not tested
Birthweight (gm)	3072±308	3065±465		
Second (treated) pregnancy				
Number	41	47	86	49
Birthweight (gm)	3268±381	3182±369	$\Delta_2 - \Delta_1 = 79$	3185±382
Females:				
First (untreated) pregnancy				
Number	64	64	79	Not tested
Birthweight (gm)	3056±364	2977±340		
Second (treated) pregnancy				
Number	40	41	113	52
Birthweight (gm)	3106±333	2993±340	$\Delta_2 - \Delta_1 = 34$	2978±388

*Taken from Herriot RM, Hsueh AM, Aitchison R: Influence of maternal diet on offspring: growth, behavior, feed efficiency, and susceptibility (human). A study in Juilian, Taiwan, initiated by Bacon F. Chow. (Mimeo: Final report to National Institutes of Child Health and Human Development, Washington, D.C.)

**Infants are included only if mothers consumed more than half the supplement given them in the last five months of pregnancy, and who were weighed within 24 hours of delivery.

The Dutch Famine Study [Stein et al, 1975]

This study is unique in that food deprivation and rehabilitation occurred in totally different circumstances from those described in any other. The affected population lived in a country in which food had been plentiful. Although for the three years of the German military occupation before the famine to which the index pregnancies were exposed, the mothers were on a low calorie diet and below their usual body weight, the diet was well-balanced and they were reported to be in a reasonably good nutritional state. During some part of pregnancy the mothers were subjected to a six-month period of near starvation followed by rapid rehabilitation. This experience is a close analogue of many animal experiments on which prevailing theories of prenatal nutritional effects are based [cf Winick and Noble, 1966; Barnes et al, 1968].

Maternities in the western Netherlands that occurred during the "hunger winter" of 1944–45 were described early on by Sindram [1945], Stroink [1947], Smith [1947], and later by others [Stein and Susser, 1975; Stein et al, 1975]. Several historical points should be noted. A measure of the available diet could be calculated from the official ration; this was published weekly for each region throughout the war and the famine. Because the famine lasted about six months, no woman was exposed for the full duration of a term pregnancy. The deprivation of food among city dwellers, while of short duration, was never less than severe and at times life-threatening. Rations provided a measure of dietary deprivation for monthly birth cohorts that can be assigned high validity because of the general shortage of food everywhere. A weakness of the study, however, was the lack of any measure of individual diets. All major analyses were therefore in terms of cohorts and not individuals.

Data on more than 6,000 consecutive maternities were collected from teaching hospital records in famine and control cities. The sharp decrease in food was accurately and immediately mirrored in the postpartum weight of the mothers. By contrast, birthweight and other infant dimensions were slower to reflect the fall-off in food and were clearly modulated by a maternal buffer. Thus, effects on infant size were seen only when a threshold level in the diet of the affected groups had been crossed. Famine effects on fetal growth were further limited in that they occurred with exposure in late pregnancy only and not with exposure in the first two trimesters. The effects on birthweight were substantial (a mean reduction of about 300 gm at the height of the famine and a maximum gain of perhaps 400 gm in the postfamine period). These effects resulted from growth retardation; the mean length of gestation was not significantly affected among groups of infants who showed famine effects.

Dynamic changes in the relations between maternal weight, placental weight and fetal dimensions were associated with semi-starvation. The size of the effects of various growth indices was concomitant with the time-order in which they became apparent. First maternal weight was affected, then birthweight, then placental weight, then length, and then head size. With prolonged starvation, it was inferred, the usual mode of nutrient transfer from mother to placenta and infant was modified. Above the nutritional threshold value and before fetal growth was affected, analysis suggests that nutrients passed into maternal stores and indirectly from maternal stores to the fetus and that fetal size determined placental size. Below the threshold value, maternal intake appeared to be transmitted directly to the fetus, and placental size became a determinant of fetal size.

Women whose exposure to famine was limited solely to the first trimester and who were suddenly restored to a normal diet at the liberation provide a possible analogy to the third-trimester supplementation of ill-nourished women. Among such women, birthweights were on the average well above those of infants born during the famine whose mothers were exposed in later pregnancy. These women may also provide an analogy to that minority of supplemented women in the New York and Montreal studies who experienced an untoward outcome. In this cohort of women, whose exposure to famine was limited to the first trimester, there was a small excess of births under 2,500 gm, an excess of stillbirths and first-day deaths, and an excess of first-week deaths attributed to prematurity. The initial hypothesis proposed in the report of the study was that these effects resulted from first-trimester famine exposure, possibly in interaction with infection. In the light of the apparently adverse effects of supplementation in a minority of women in the New York and Montreal studies, however, an adverse effect of supplementation in a minority of undernourished women cannot be ruled out as the explanation.

On the other hand, the Dutch study provides unequivocal evidence that severe prenatal nutritional deprivation in the latter part of pregnancy not only retards fetal growth but also contributes substantially to mortality through the first three months of life, especially after the first week. In large part, this mortality was mediated through fetal growth retardation. Fortunately, the young adult male survivors of intrauterine famine exposure were in most aspects indistinguishable from control cohorts in mental, physical and health status. There were no detectable effects of exposure in late pregnancy on young adults except diminution in the frequency of obesity. Exposure early in pregnancy was associated with a small excess of defects of the central nervous system and also with an excess in the frequency of obesity [Ravelli, Stein, and Susser, 1976].

These ultimate physical and psychological outcomes, like mortality, were measured in about 120,000 19-year-old urban-born men at standardized military induction medical examinations. The men were subjected to a battery of cognitive tests of which Raven's Progressive Matrices were the most sensitive. Since the degree and timing of the famine and the available food rations were well documented, intrauterine exposure could be deduced from place and date of birth. About 40,000 men had been exposed during gestation.

Several alternatives to a null hypothesis might be advanced to explain the absence of detectable effects. The most plausible is that brain growth was affected — head size at birth was reduced in those exposed in late pregnancy — but not to a degree that would affect function. Dobbing and Sands [1973] have demonstrated a continuing brain growth spurt well into the second year of life; prenatal deprivation would therefore comprise only about 10% of the hypothesized vulnerable period. It could also be that effects were present early in life, but were overwhelmed by the predominant influence of the postnatal environment. The likelihood of early effects, for the usual tests of cognition, is diminished by the results of the New York study. Still another possibility is that unmeasured mental functions were affected. The likelihood that some effects went undetected because unmeasured is raised by the findings on habituation, dishabituation, and play in the New York study.

We therefore restrict our conclusions from the Dutch famine study to the prevailing socioeconomic and nutritional conditions, to prenatal exposure, and to conventional psychometric measures. We are then safe in saying that in economically developed societies, exposure even to severe prenatal deprivation will leave no mark on conventional measures of cognitive function.

CONCLUSIONS

Birthweight

The new generation of studies of the past decade moves us somewhat closer to securing causal inferences about the effects of prenatal nutrition in free-living human beings. From them we conclude that, among women at risk of producing low birthweight infants, prenatal dietary supplements can lead to modest rise in birthweight, say about 40 to 70 gm. The degree of the rise seems to be conditional and to depend on the nutritional state of the woman. In thin or undernourished women the rise in birthweight can be expected to be in the upper range. In heavier women there is unlikely to be any rise. In starved women a deficit of about 300 gm can be made up immediately upon restoring normal diet in the latter half of pregnancy. Other results support the notion of conditional effects of deprivation and supplementation. In the Dutch famine study variation in food availability in a population on a well-balanced, if sparse, diet bore no relation to fetal growth until there was severe food deprivation. In the New York experiment, prenatal diet supplements appeared to protect against fetal growth retardation under the specific condition that mothers were heavy cigarette smokers.

A high protein diet (in combination with low calorie intake) has proved harmful to some women. This phenomenon occurred in circumstances where there was no protein deficiency in the regular diet. In two studies diet supplementation appeared as an especial hazard for women with prior low birthweight deliveries, but note that in one of these, the Montreal study, the protein content is not known to us. Studies of nutritional supplements in food-deprived rhesus monkeys give indications of similar results [Riopelle and Favrett, 1977; Riopelle and Hale, 1975; Riopelle, Hale and Watts, 1976; Riopelle, Hill, and Li, 1975]. Thus, animals on high protein supplements gave birth prematurely. There was no growth retardation of the infants, as there was in the New York study, and infant mortality seemed to be influenced favorably. On the other hand, the high protein supplement induced maternal weight gain that was not transmuted into birthweight, a finding similar to that of the New York study. Although based on much smaller numbers than the human study, the results of this primate study gain from control and precision in experimental application.

Protein has seemed no more effective than calories in raising birthweight. In Bogotá a relatively high protein food supplement was used, but there is no way of telling whether calories alone would have produced an effect. In Guatemala, birthweight in protein-supplemented villages was no higher than in calorie-supplemented villages. In the New York study, both high protein and balanced supplements protected against the ill effects of heavy smoking, partially in the case of maternal weight gain and completely in the case of birthweight.

In other respects, however, the two supplements produced different effects. Thus there were effects of the high protein Supplement on maternal weight gain, but these were not reflected in placental or fetal growth and were adverse in a small group of women. By contrast, there were no significant effects of the balanced Complement on maternal weight gain, while there were effects on the placental biochemistry. Thus the analysis of placental biochemistry in the New York study gives indications, not reported here, of specific action of nutritional supplements that depend on the precise make-up and balance of the component nutrients. The results give added weight to studies of the associations of specific nutrients with birthweight and other measures of birth outcome [Crosby et al, 1977; Metcoff, 1978]. These associations will need to be tested in further experimental studies in animals, and with due caution, in pregnant women. With regard to the timing of nutritional intervention, the results obtained have been produced, in most studies, by supplementation or deprivation confined to the latter half of pregnancy. The Guatemala researchers, however, argue from their analysis that if supplementation were begun earlier and sustained throughout gestation, the effects would be additive. As presented, the analysis is not conclusive.

Among the many questions about prenatal nutrition and fetal growth that require fresh study are the following:

Under what conditions, if any, does protein have a place in dietary intervention in the prenatal period?

If high protein dietary supplementation is harmful to women at high risk of premature births because of a history of such births, what are the implications for prenatal care? And what may this result indicate about the causes of premature births?

What are the effects likely to be of dietary supplementation with specific nutrients tailored to specific needs? Challenging issues of research design are posed by the descriptive and exploratory studies carried out so far.

Are males truly more sensitive to intrauterine nutritional deficiencies than females? Exploration of the interactions between specific characteristics of mother and fetus may yield new insights.

What factors (other than genetic) account for the substantial differences in size at birth in the United States among social classes, ethnic groups, and races? The results reported here plainly indicate that nutrition alone cannot explain them.

Psychological Effects

The data refer mainly to four studies of prenatal nutrition, that is, the Dutch, New York, Guatemala, and Taiwan studies. In the Dutch famine a previously well-nourished population, when exposed to prenatal deprivation of nutrients below a threshold value during the third trimester of pregnancy, showed unequivocal effects of depressed fertility, retarded fetal growth, and increased mortality up to three months of age. Yet among adult male survivors no effects of exposure in late pregnancy could be detected except in the frequency of obesity. Their cognitive abilities were unimpaired on a battery of tests. These tests were sensitive to a range of subtle demographic indices (birth rank, family size, maternal age) but not to intrauterine famine exposure.

In the New York study, the population was at high risk of low birthweight, but only segments of it could be described as poorly nourished. In this population, prenatal supplementation significantly benefited growth under the smoking condition only. Nonetheless, the high protein Supplement benefited performance on specific psychological tests. This benefit, while unconditional, was not mediated by fetal growth. The positive "protein-related" responses were in turn unrelated to the more usual infant psychological tests (which themselves were "growth related" in that they correlated with fetal and infant growth).

The published data of the Guatemala study afford some reassurance with regard to supplementation. In this instance, the total population suffered from chronic undernutrition, and hence the favorable effects observed on fetal growth and later test performance are subject to that condition. Even within this population, however, the results were conditional, and increments in fetal growth were most notable among women most likely to be malnourished. The same was true of mental performance, although in this domain postnatal as well as prenatal factors were involved.

The Taiwan study of women on a marginal low protein diet and given a substantial supplement of protein and calories yielded results that were not statistically significant. For birthweight the results were of the same order of magnitude as in all the other studies reviewed here. Psychological effects, if present, were unremarkable. Although the study was closely monitored, numbers were small and the analysis undermined by potential self-selection of those included.

Taking together the data available to us on the *usual measures* we conclude that severe prenatal nutritional deprivation, in the presence of good nutritional and social conditions in the postnatal environment, is unlikely to affect cognitive function in adults. This conclusion excepts certain measures of mental function that are not growth related, especially habituation.

The evidence that early postnatal environment affects cognitive competence is strong indeed; its influence seems likely to overwhelm small nutritional effects. Two well-designed and well-executed experimental studies [Garber, 1975; McKay et al, 1976], as well as other quasi-experimental and observational studies [Skodak and Skeels, 1945; Record, McKeown and

Edwards, 1969b; Belmont and Marolla, 1973; Belmont, Stein and Susser, 1975], make this a conclusion hardly open to challenge. Among such postnatal environmental influences on cognitive competence, the part of nutrition seems to be well supported by the Guatemala study. Other studies of early postnatal malnutrition have also detected adverse effects at follow-up [Hertzig et al, 1972; Richardson, 1976], although similar studies have failed to do so [Hansen et al, 1971].

For overt chronic malnutrition extending into the prenatal period, critical pieces of the puzzle are still missing. It is possible, but not established, that prenatal malnutrition contributes to early deficiencies in the usual measures of cognitive competence. Such effects might be present early in life and disappear later, or might persist only in the presence of chronic postnatal undernutrition.

Even the Guatemala study does not show effects on cognition solely attributable to prenatal nutrition. Thus on the simplest interpretation the most that can be concluded from the Guatemala reports is that some combination of prenatal nutrition with the postnatal environment influences early cognitive function. A less obvious interpretation may be that the reported associations of prenatal nutrition with early cognitive function are solely attributable to the social environment and the postnatal nutrition of the child. In other words, the data from existing studies do not exclude the possibility that a harsh social environment is the common cause both of malnutrition and of retarded performance on the usual cognitive measures, outcomes separate but conflated by their common origin.

In this respect, one may advance a hypothetical model to encompass the work of Chavez and Martinez [1975] and Cravioto and Delicardie [1975] in Mexico, of Hertzig et al [1972] and Richardson [1976] in Jamaica, and of Hansen et al [1971] in South Africa, as well as the animal experiments of Frankova [1974, 1978] and others.

The work of Chavez underlines the importance of the nutritional state on affect and behavior. His baseline observations began with a small cohort of mothers and their infants in a poor and remote Mexican village. He then instituted continuous supplementation of diet during the subsequent pregnancies of mothers and their later-born infants. The offspring of the later, supplemented cohort were distinctly larger and livelier than the first. The advantage in performance of the better-nourished cohort seemed to the observer to stem from the stimulus they gave to their parents, who were much more reactive and attentive to them than they had been to their older sibs. The nutritional intervention thus set off a cycle of reciprocal interaction. In this interaction the physical state of the child and the affective state of the mother (responsive both to her nutritional state and the behavior of the child) evidently played an important part. From this work we can draw no firm conclusion about the direct effect of prenatal nutrition on the child's mental performance.

The work of Cravioto points to the importance of social stimulation in countering the effects of poverty and poor nutrition on mental performance. In another poor Mexican village, he conducted over many years a much larger study than that of Chavez. Cravioto and DeLicardie [1975] found (as hypothesized) that depressed growth and mental performance were associated with poor maternal and child nutrition. In comparisons of families closely matched for socioeconomic status, however, the association with nutrition disappeared, and the only factor that then discriminated between the mental performance of the children was social stimulation; to be precise, the mother's radio listening. Hence, we can not attribute effects solely to nutrition, either prenatal or postnatal.

Richardson [1976] found that between social stimulation and early malnutrition there was interaction, the one reinforcing the other. In a Jamaican follow-up study of boys who had been admitted to a hospital for acute nutritional failure (kwashiorkor) in the first two years of life, Hertzig et al [1972] had found depressed mental performance at pubescence when compared with sibs and neighborhood controls. The retardation occurred only among the rural and not among the urban dwellers. Richardson later found that a great part of the difference could be explained by a measure of intrafamilial social stimulation. Lack of stimulation appeared to exacerbate the effects of early malnutrition. In the absence of evidence it is of course possible, as the work of Chavez suggests, that a child passive as a result of malnutrition failed to elicit stimulation from his parents, and that this passivity was the common cause of the association of depressed cognitive performance with both lack of social stimulation and early malnutrition. In a similar study in Cape Town, Hansen, and colleagues [Hansen et al, 1971] failed to find a difference in cognitive performance between cases of early kwashiorkor and their sibs at 10 years of age. If there had been an effect at earlier ages, it must have been reversed by that time.

In an elegant series of animal experiments on nutritional deprivation and development Frankova has shown how subtle are the effects of the social environment, and how difficult to control. Malnutrition of the dam damped her responsiveness to the litter, and the development of her offspring. Alternative sources of social stimulation — for instance provided by castrated "aunts" or surrogate mothers — counteracted these depressing effects [Frankova 1974, 1978].

This work on postnatal nutrition taken together suggests that under conditions of chronic malnutrition, postnatal nutritional state influences current affective state and somatic growth. Its influence on psychological test performance will be in interaction with the social environment. The data also suggest that diet supplementation improves the affective state and activity of a malnourished mother, as well as of the offspring. This maternal effect in turn is a likely intermediate variable in a path leading from nutrition of the mother through affect of the mother to improvement in the psychological performance of the offspring.

The hypothesis of Klein et al [1978] is that in Guatemala prenatal as well as postnatal nutritional supplementation improved psychological test performance, but this hypothesis has not yet been adequately tested in their data. On the basis of the above, another tenable hypothesis could be that improvements in the mother's health and affective state improve child care and stimulation and consequently the child's growth and development.

These several effects of nutrition (on the postnatal somatic growth of the child, on the prenatal and postnatal physical and mental state of the mother) are likely to interact in complex and reciprocal fashion with the mental performance of the child. This hypothetical process can be illustrated in a path diagram:

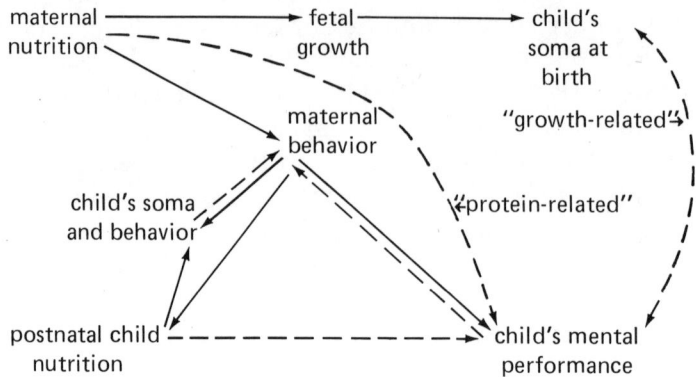

The path from fetal growth to mental performance is omitted in favor of the noncommittal association — without causal direction — between the child's somatic and mental performance. Still another generation of studies will be required to separate out the contribution of these factors and their interactions and to establish causal pathways.

The New York study data on the protein-related psychological measures require separate interpretation from the more usual "growth-related" measures. We noted, in the New York study, that one-year-old infants of mothers who took the high protein Supplement during pregnancy exhibited more rapid visual habituation, brisker dishabituation, and longer episodes of play with toys, than did infants in the other two treatment groups. In Chapter IV we suggested that the direction of these responses was favorable, although their significance for mental performance at later ages is far from clear. Data on habituation from a study of primates [Boelkins and Hegsted, 1978], as well as the observation from the Bogotá study in early postnatal life [Mora et al, 1979] also bear on these results. While experimental conditions and age at testing varied greatly, the results can be taken as concordant with those of the New York study.

The true significance of these various results is as yet obscure. They too must await another generation of studies to establish their meaning. Yet as we observed in closing Chapter IV, the results of our New York study have created a painful dilemma for those who would apply high protein prenatal treatments. The apparent physical risks of the high protein supplement may be balanced by the apparent psychological benefits. In view of the seeming dangers, the best path to follow at this time, we believe, is through the observational approach and through animal studies. The testing and elaboration of the results by such approaches may permit the resumption of human intervention studies at some later stage.

To the outstanding questions raised above, in concluding our discussion on prenatal nutrition with fetal growth as an outcome, we must then add other questions with psychological development as an outcome:

With regard to the usual "growth-related" measures of psychological development.

Does prenatal nutrition as a sole factor affect these measures, if not in the developed world, even in the chronically malnourished populations of the less developed world? If it does, what is the size of its contribution?

Does prenatal nutrition interact with social environmental factors to affect these measures? If it does, what precisely are the factors with which prenatal nutrition interacts? Is the size of its contribution, if any, large enough to give rise to concern for its effects on these aspects of development?

With regard to the "protein-related" measures of psychological development.

Can their relationship to prenatal protein diet be confirmed in other studies, in animal experiments, or from less direct evidence?

If the findings are replicated, how early in development might differences in these measures appear?

What do these measures at one year of age signify for later psychological development?

Might the favorable one-year-old outcome produced by a high protein supplement in the New York study be attained by a lesser protein boost in chronically malnourished populations of less developed countries? And might the risk of an adverse effect, if it exists in such populations, be thereby averted?

We conclude that we must accept less ambitious and more specific objectives for prenatal nutrition programs, in all the forms tried so far, than when the present generation of studies began. We can expect that prenatal energy supplements will produce modest increments in fetal growth under appropriate conditions. Similarly we can expect that such supplements will improve perinatal and early postnatal mortality (although, excepting the recovery from the Dutch famine, no study has had the statistical power for conclusive demonstration). We can expect also that a program of prenatal and postnatal supplementation and medical care will, as in the Guatemala study, improve both physical growth and cognitive performance (although we do not know what prenatal supplementation alone will do).

Appendices

APPENDIX 1.1. Information Collected on Participants During Pregnancy

Category	Description
Historical:	
Medical and obstetric	Past pregnancy experience; weight at conception; smoking; history of diabetes, hypertension, toxemia, infection, other renal disease, and narcotic or heavy alcohol use (grounds for exclusion or discontinuation in the study). Changes in above variables during gestation.
Social, demographic, and economic	Occupational status of participant, participant's father and spouse; work during pregnancy; income; education; type and adequacy of housing; family structure; geographic and occupational mobility; income; public assistance; marital status.
Nutritional	Quantitative 24-hour diet recall at recruitment and three further times during the remainder of gestation; adherence to supplements; status of appetite; presence of nausea or vomiting; other diet changes. Urinary riboflavin excretion.
Psychological	Items from protocols of Langner et al [1970].
Physical:	
Anthropometric	Weight (serially) and height, arm circumference, and skinfold thickness (triceps and subscapular), at recruitment.
Medical and obstetric	Serial blood pressure, uterine size, general course of pregnancy.
Biochemical:	
Nutritional	1. Hematocrit. 2. Vitamins A, B_6, and ascorbic acid, in serum at registration and delivery. 3. Serum taken at registration and delivery was stored for later use.*
Urine riboflavin	To corroborate history of adherence to supplements, at all clinic visits.
Immunologic:	Specific antibody determinations on stored maternal sera taken at registration and delivery, and on cord blood when infant IgM levels were high.

*Many of the sera that were drawn at registration and delivery were lost during storage following failures of power to our freezers.

APPENDIX 1.2. Information Collected on Participants at Delivery and Follow-Up

Category	Description
Historical:	
Medical and obstetric	Medical events at delivery and during the first year of life, including history of infection, use of medical services, immunization status.
Socioeconomic	Changes from initial history.
Nutritional	Intake of infant in hospital; quantitative 24-hour diet recall at 6 to 8 weeks of age and at about one year of age; general infant feeding behavior.
From direct examination of infant:	
Anthropometric	Weight at birth, during the hospital stay, at 6 to 8 weeks, and at one year; length at birth, 6 to 8 weeks, and at one year; head circumference and diameters at birth, at 6 to 8 weeks, and at one year; arm circumference and subscapular and triceps skinfold thickness at birth and at one year.
General and neurologic	Apgar score; physical and neurologic indices of maturity at birth; neurologic screening at one year.
Psychodevelopmental	Neonatal: lateralization; habituation to sound and tactile stimuli; structured observation of behavior and activity level; visual pursuit.
	At one year of age: developmental examination; habituation to visual stimuli; object retention; structured observation of open field play and interaction with mother.
Anatomic, gross and microscopic:	
Umbilical cord	Microscopic examination, and histomorphometry.
Placenta	Weight; gross and microscopic examination; histomorphometry.
Biochemical:	DNA, RNA, protein and alkaline ribonuclease content of the placenta.
Immunologic:	Infant IgM levels on the third day of life; cord and mother's sera if infant's 3-day IgM elevated.

APPENDIX 2.1. Three Indices of Weight Gain by Treatment and Entry Cohort: a. All deliveries

Total deliveries	Supplement	Complement	Control	Total
Stage of gestation at registration (weeks):				
1. Total weight gain (lbs)				
<15	24.9* ± 10.3 (78)	23.1 ± 10.7 (93)	21.8* ± 9.9 (108)	23.1 ± 10.4 (279)
15–19	23.8 ± 10.9 (66)	25.6 ± 13.5 (57)	22.0 ± 12.7 (66)	23.7 ± 12.5 (189)
20–24	23.7 ± 12.6 (52)	21.9 ± 12.3 (59)	22.0 ± 13.7 (46)	22.5 ± 12.8 (157)
25+	18.0* ± 11.0 (39)	23.0* ± 7.8 (35)	19.9 ± 14.2 (33)	20.2 ± 11.4 (107)
Total	23.3 ± 11.3 (239)	23.4 ± 11.5 (245)	21.6 ± 12.0 (256)	22.7 ± 11.7 (740)
2. Average weight gain (lbs/wk)				
<15	0.91* ± 0.46 (78)	0.92* ± 0.32 (94)	0.83* ± 0.32 (108)	0.88 ± 0.37 (280)
15–19	1.05 ± 0.49 (66)	0.94 ± 0.46 (57)	0.96 ± 0.42 (66)	0.99 ± 0.46 (189)
20–24	0.98 ± 0.47 (53)	0.93 ± 0.53 (58)	0.98[a] ± 0.54 (46)	0.96[a] ± 0.52 (157)
25+	0.87 ± 0.62 (39)	1.03 ± 0.52 (36)	0.96[a] ± 0.59 (32)	0.95[a] ± 0.58 (107)
Total	0.96 ± 0.50 (240)	0.95 ± 0.44 (246)	0.91 ± 0.45 (255)	0.94 ± 0.46 (741)
3. Early weight gain (lbs/wk)				
<15	0.84* ± 0.58 (71)	0.71 ± 0.67 (80)	0.60* ± 0.66 (93)	0.71 ± 0.65 (244)
15–19	1.08 ± 0.67 (59)	0.99 ± 0.66 (52)	1.02 ± 0.60 (61)	1.03 ± 0.65 (172)
20–24	1.03 ± 0.70 (43)	0.98 ± 0.81 (50)	0.97 ± 1.05 (44)	0.99 ± 0.86 (137)
25+	1.06 ± 0.73 (35)	0.99 ± 0.60 (30)	1.07 ± 0.71 (24)	1.04 ± 0.69 (89)
Total	0.99 ± 0.66 (211)	0.89 ± 0.71 (213)	0.85* ± 0.77 (225)	0.91* ± 0.72 (649)

Eight cases deviant for birthweight by gestation included in Total rows only.
[a]Two extreme outliers omitted from table. Both in Control group: +4.84 lbs/wk (37+ wk gest) and −3.83 lbs/wk (<37 wk gest).
*Significant difference in row ($p < 0.05$). ( ) = n; ± = SD.

APPENDIX 2.1 Three Indices of Weight Gain by Treatment and Entry Cohort: b. Deliveries < 37 weeks gestation

Total deliveries	Supplement	Complement	Control	Total
Stage of gestation at registration (weeks):				
1. Total weight gain (lbs)				
<15	17.7 ± 9.2 (15)	19.1 ± 10.4 (19)	22.9 ± 6.6 (19)	20.1 ± 9.1 (53)
15–19	19.9 ± 6.6 (18)	17.6 ± 4.9 (5)	17.3 ± 12.5 (22)	18.4 ± 9.9 (45)
20–24	14.4 ± 13.3 (10)	11.3 ± 7.5 (10)	14.8 ± 13.1 (12)	13.6 ± 11.8 (32)
25+	11.0 ± 5.6 (8)	24.1 ± 5.9 (7)	8.3 ± 10.0 (9)	13.8 ± 10.2 (24)
Total	16.8 ± 9.5 (51)	17.9 ± 9.5 (41)	17.3 ± 11.8 (62)	17.3 ± 10.5 (154)
2. Average weight gain (lbs/wk)				
<15	0.65 ± 0.71 (15)	0.92 ± 0.33 (19)	0.89 ± 0.33 (19)	0.83 ± 0.48 (53)
15–19	0.97 ± 0.46 (18)	0.70 ± 0.36 (5)	0.92 ± 0.53 (22)	0.92 ± 0.53 (22)
20–24	0.99 ± 0.87 (9)	0.66 ± 0.84 (10)	0.98[a] ± 0.72 (11)	0.88[a] ± 0.82 (30)
25+	0.52 ± 0.87 (8)	1.55 ± 0.62 (7)	0.83 ± 0.84 (9)	0.93 ± 0.89 (24)
Total	0.80 ± 0.72 (50)	0.94 ± 0.63 (41)	0.91[a] ± 0.58 (61)	0.88[a] ± 0.64 (152)
3. Early weight gain (lbs/wk)				
<15	0.95 ± 0.50 (13)	0.89 ± 0.93 (17)	0.79 ± 0.59 (14)	0.88 ± 0.72 (44)
15–19	0.95 ± 0.65 (17)	0.53 ± 0.77 (5)	1.11 ± 0.62 (20)	0.98 ± 0.67 (42)
20–24	0.95 ± 1.02 (8)	0.68 ± 1.10 (8)	0.52 ± 1.71 (12)	0.69 ± 1.39 (28)
25+	0.90 ± 0.73 (7)	1.47 ± 0.24 (4)	1.65 ± 0.86 (5)	1.27 ± 0.77 (16)
Total	0.94 ± 0.71 (45)	0.86 ± 0.93 (34)	0.93 ± 1.06 (51)	0.92 ± 0.92 (130)

Eight cases deviant for birthweight by gestation omitted.
[a]Two extreme outliers omitted from table. Both in Control group: +4.84 lbs/wk (37+ wk gest) and −3.83 lbs/wk (<37 wk gest).

APPENDIX 2.1 Three Indices of Weight Gain by Treatment and Entry Cohort: c. Deliveries 37+ weeks gestation

Total deliveries Stage of gestation at registration (weeks):	Supplement	Complement	Control	Total
1. Total weight gain (lbs)				
<15	26.6* ± 9.9 (63)	24.2 ± 10.5 (74)	21.5* ± 10.4 (89)	23.8 ± 10.5 (226)
15–19	25.2 ± 11.9 (48)	26.4 ± 13.8 (52)	24.3 ± 12.2 (44)	25.4 ± 12.7 (144)
20–24	25.9 ± 11.3 (42)	24.0 ± 11.9 (49)	24.5 ± 12.9 (34)	24.8 ± 12.0 (125)
25+	19.8 ± 11.3 (31)	22.8 ± 8.1 (28)	24.2 ± 13.0 (24)	22.1 ± 11.1 (83)
Total	24.9 ± 11.2 (184)	24.5 ± 11.6 (203)	23.0 ± 11.8 (191)	24.2 ± 11.6 (578)
2. Average weight gain (lbs/wk)				
<15	0.98* ± 0.36 (63)	0.92 ± 0.32 (75)	0.81* ± 0.32 (89)	0.90 ± 0.34 (227)
15–19	1.08 ± 0.50 (48)	0.97 ± 0.46 (52)	0.99 ± 0.36 (44)	0.45 ± 0.45 (144)
20–24	0.98 ± 0.33 (44)	0.99 ± 0.42 (48)	0.98 ± 0.47 (35)	0.98 ± 0.41 (127)
25+	0.96 ± 0.49 (31)	0.90 ± 0.40 (29)	1.01[a] ± 0.45 (23)	0.95[a] ± 0.45 (83)
Total	1.00 ± 0.42 (186)	0.95 ± 0.40 (204)	0.91[a] ± 0.39 (191)	0.95[a] ± 0.40 (581)
3. Early weight gain (lbs/wk)				
<15	0.82* ± 0.59 (58)	0.67 ± 0.58 (63)	0.57* ± 0.66 (79)	0.67 ± 0.62 (200)
15–19	1.14 ± 0.67 (42)	1.04 ± 0.63 (47)	0.98 ± 0.59 (41)	1.05 ± 0.64 (130)
20–24	1.04 ± 0.61 (35)	1.04 ± 0.73 (42)	1.14 ± 0.55 (32)	1.07 ± 0.64 (109)
25+	1.10 ± 0.73 (28)	0.92 ± 0.61 (26)	0.92 ± 0.57 (19)	0.99 ± 0.65 (73)
Total	1.00* ± 0.66 (163)	0.89 ± 0.66 (178)	0.81 ± 0.66 (171)	0.90 ± 0.66 (512)

Eight cases deviant for birthweight by gestation omitted.
[a]Two extreme outliers omitted from table. Both in Control group: +4.84 lbs/wk (37+ wk gest) and −3.83 lbs/wk (<37 wk gest).
*Significant difference in row ($p < 0.05$). ( ) = n; ± = SD.

APPENDIX 2.2a. Early Weight Gain and Treatment: Multiple regression analysis

Step in multiple regression analysis	Variable	Regression coefficient (B); lbs/wk × 100	F value for regression coefficient	Change in R^2 at entry	F value for change in R^2
1	Parity (n)	−0.76	0.10	0.002	1.03
2	Past low bw infants (n)	3.66	0.44	0.001	0.88
3	Cigarettes/d, at registration (n)	−0.94	6.56	0.008	4.99
4	Weight at conception (lbs)	−0.20	0.25	0.006	3.87
5	Stage gestation at registration (d)	0.36	23.57	0.041	27.84
6	Weight at registration (lbs)	−0.21	0.32	0.001	0.65
7	[a]Initial diet recall not completed = 1, others = 0	14.25	0.91	0.000	0.02
8	Protein intake, 24 hrs prior to registration (gm)	0.22	8.34	0.012	8.49
9	Supplement = 1, others = 0	11.72	2.97	0.005	3.21
10	Complement = 1, others = 0	2.23	0.11	0.000	0.11

Stepwise multiple regression analysis with early weight gain (lbs/wk) as dependent variable, and several variables including treatment group as independent variables (n = 641 mothers of singleton infants with known dependent variable; 8 cases with birthweight deviant for gestation omitted.) Constant = 79.19.

[a]n = 26.

R = multiple correlation.

Change in R^2 at entry is the change in variance associated with variable entered at that step in analysis controlling for all variables previously entered.

F at entry = F value associated with the variable, controlling for all variables previously entered.

$p = 0.05$, $F = 3.84$; $p = 0.01$, $F = 6.63$; $p = 0.001$, $F = 10.83$.

APPENDIX 2.2b. Early Weight Gain and Treatment: Multiple regression analysis

Step in multiple regression analysis	Variable	Regression coefficient (B); lbs/wk × 100	F value for regression coefficient	change in R^2 at entry	F value for change in R^2
1	Parity (n)	3.43	1.04	0.002	1.03
2	Past low bw infants (n)	−12.46	2.13	0.001	0.88
3	Cigarettes/d, at registration (n)	−0.93	6.43	0.008	4.99
4	Weight at conception (lbs)	−0.22	0.31	0.006	3.87
5	Stage gestation at registration (d)	0.36	24.40	0.041	27.84
6	Weight at registration (lbs)	−0.20	0.28	0.001	0.65
7	[a]Initial diet recall not completed = 1, others = 0	16.46	1.20	0.000	0.02
8	Protein intake, 24 hours prior to registration (gm)	0.24	9.30	0.012	8.49
9	Supplement = 1, others = 0	10.95	1.77	0.005	3.21
10	Complement = 1, others = 0	6.75	0.68	0.000	0.11
11	1 × 9	−4.01	0.44	0.000	0.25
12	2 × 9	22.50	2.60	0.001	0.48
13	1 × 10	−11.79	4.30	0.001	0.71
14	2 × 10	31.06	6.33	0.009	6.33

Stepwise multiple regression analysis with early weight gain (lbs/wk) as dependent variable and several variables including treatment group as independent variables (n = 641 mothers of singleton infants with known dependent variable; 8 cases with birthweight deviant for gestation omitted. Constant = 78.22.
[a]n = 26.
R = multiple correlation.
Change in R^2 at entry is the change in variance associated with variable entered at that step in analysis controlling for all variables previously entered.
F at entry = F value associated with the variable, controlling for all variables previously entered.
p = 0.05, F = 3.84; p = 0.01, F = 6.63; p = 0.001, F = 10.83.

APPENDIX 2.2c. Average Weight Gain and Treatment: Multiple regression analysis

Step in multiple regression analysis	Variable	Regression coefficient (B); lbs/wk × 100	F value for regression coefficient	Change in R^2 at entry	F value for change in R^2
1	Parity (n)	−2.56	3.05	0.018	13.45
2	Past low bw infants (n)	−4.63	1.99	0.003	2.54
3	Cigarettes/d, at registration (n)	−0.66	8.32	0.009	6.97
4	Weight at conception (lbs)	0.15	0.39	1.000	0.01
5	Stage of gestation at registration (d)	0.11	5.78	0.008	5.96
6	Weight at registration (lbs)	−0.15	0.49	0.001	0.56
7	[a]Initial diet recall not completed = 1, others = 0	4.89	0.31	0.000	0.05
8	Protein intake, 24 hours prior to registration (gm)	0.05	1.30	0.002	1.49
9	Supplement = 1, others = 0	4.01	0.92	0.001	0.38
10	Complement = 1, others = 0	3.56	0.74	0.001	0.74

Stepwise multiple regression analysis with average weight gain (lbs/wk) as dependent variable and several variables including treatment group as independent variables (n = 732 mothers of singleton infants with known dependent variable; 8 cases with birthweight deviant for gestation omitted). Constant = 84.23.

[a]n = 33.

R = multiple correlation.

Change in the R^2 at entry is the change in variance associated with variable entered at that step in analysis controlling for all variables previously entered.

F at entry = F value associated with the variable, controlling for all variables previously entered.

$p = 0.05$, F = 3.84; $p = 0.01$, F = 6.63; $p = 0.001$, F = 10.83.

APPENDIX 2.2d. Average Weight Gain and Treatment: Multiple regression analysis

Step in multiple regression analysis	Variable	Regression coefficient (B): lbs/wk × 100	F value for regression coefficient	Change in R^2 at entry	F value for change in R^2
1	Parity (n)	-2.98	2.04	0.018	13.45
2	Past low bw infants (n)	-1.61	0.09	0.003	2.54
3	Cigarettes/d, at registration (n)	-1.09	5.99	0.009	6.97
4	Weight at conception (lbs)	0.55	1.95	0.000	0.01
5	Stage gestation at registration (d)	0.16	4.34	0.008	5.96
6	Weight at registration (lbs)	-0.10	0.08	0.001	0.56
7	[a]Initial diet recall not completed = 1, others = 0	5.38	0.37	0.000	0.05
8	Protein intake, 24 hours prior to registration (gm)	0.05	1.05	0.002	1.49
9	Supplement = 1, others = 0	86.68	4.69	0.001	0.38
10	Complement = 1, others = 0	93.70	5.42	0.001	0.74
11	1 × 9	1.70	0.21	0.000	0.16
12	2 × 9	-2.22	0.07	0.000	0.01
13	1 × 10	-0.52	0.02	0.000	0.18
14	2 × 10	-5.70	0.37	0.000	0.07
15	3 × 9	0.24	0.26	0.000	0.15
16	3 × 10	0.77	1.70	0.002	1.44
17	4 × 9	-0.14	0.06	0.001	0.64
18	5 × 9	-0.09	0.62	0.002	1.37
19	6 × 9	-0.48	0.78	0.002	1.52
20	4 × 10	-1.01	2.90	0.007	5.30
21	5 × 10	-0.07	0.46	0.000	0.25
22	6 × 10	0.28	0.25	0.000	0.25

Stepwise multiple regression analysis with average weight gain (lbs/wk) as dependent variable and several variables including treatment group as independent variables (n = 732 mothers of singletons with known dependent variable; 8 cases with birthweight deviant for gestation omitted). Constant = 25.04.

Constant 25.04.

[a]n = 33.

R = multiple correlation.

Change in R^2 at entry is the change in variance associated with variable entered at that step in analysis controlling for all variables previously entered.

F at entry = F value associated with the variable, controlling for all variables previously entered.

$p = 0.05, F = 3.84; p = 0.01, F = 6.63; p = 0.001, F = 10.83$.

APPENDIX 2.2e. Average Weight Gain and Diet Intake: Multiple regression analysis

Step in multiple regression analysis	Variable	Regression coefficient (B); lbs/wk × 100	F value for regression coefficient	Change in R^2 at entry	F value for change in R^2
1	Parity (n)	−2.70	3.41	0.018	13.45
2	Past low bw infants (n)	−4.59	1.97	0.003	2.54
3	Cigarettes/d, at registration	−0.67	8.50	0.009	6.97
4	Weight at conception (lbs)	0.10	0.18	0.000	0.01
5	Stage gestation at registration	0.11	6.40	0.008	5.96
6	Weight at registration (lbs)	−0.12	0.28	0.001	0.56
7	[a]Initial diet recall not completed = 1, others = 0	8.23	0.86	0.000	0.05
8	Protein intake, 24 hrs prior to registration (gm)	0.03	0.41	0.002	1.49
9	[b]No data, diet intake during study = 1, others = 0	−1.29	0.02	0.005	3.66
10	Average calories/day during study	0.0015	0.14	0.006	4.20
11	Average protein/day during study (gm)	0.10	1.33	0.002	1.33

Stepwise multiple regression analysis with average weight gain as dependent variable, and several independent variables, including calorie and protein intake reported during study (n = 732 mothers of singletons with known dependent variables; 8 cases with birthweight deviant for gestation omitted). Constant = 75.42.
[a]n = 33.
[b]n = 48.
R = multiple correlation.
Change in R^2 at entry is the change in variance associated with variable entered at that step in analysis controlling for all variables previously entered.
F at entry = F value, associated with the variable, controlling for all variables previously entered.
$p = 0.05$, F = 3.84; $p = 0.01$, F = 6.63; $p = 0.001$, F = 10.83.

APPENDIX 3.1. Treatment and Prematurity: Life table analysis

Completed weeks gestation	Supplement vs controls	Supplement vs complement	Supplement vs remainder	Complement vs controls	Complement vs remainder
20	0.01	0.59	0.05	0.76	0.71
21	0.21	0.02	0.04	0.14	0.00
22	0.00	0.05	0.03	0.08	0.00
23	0.11	0.05	0.31	0.08	0.04
24	0.11	0.05	0.31	0.08	0.04
25	0.00	0.03	0.03	0.01	0.00
26	0.23	0.03	0.82	0.01	0.44
27	0.18	0.01	0.68	0.02	0.41
28	0.36	0.01	1.38	0.14	1.02
29	0.57	0.18	2.24	0.38	1.80
30	1.61	0.39	3.51	0.03	1.39
31	0.77	0.00	1.57	0.00	0.52
32	0.69	0.00	1.42	0.00	0.49
33	1.86	0.32	3.04	0.02	0.72
34	0.49	0.07	1.21	0.04	0.63
35	0.00	0.00	0.16	0.60	1.89
36	0.05	0.74	0.41	3.14	3.60
37	0.29	0.09	0.02	2.17	1.95
38	1.19	0.00	3.28	2.16	1.20
39	1.04	0.00	2.62	2.39	1.55
40	1.27	0.02	1.89	2.92	2.01
41	2.05	0.00	0.80	2.86	1.56
42	0.03	0.02	0.66	0.13	1.50
43	0.01	0.00	1.13	0.26	2.20
44	0.01	0.00	1.16	0.13	1.98

χ^2 values for comparisons of cumulative delivery rate among life tables of treatment groups, including all participants in treatment at each stage of gestation excepting 8 cases deviant for length of gestation by birthweight, and counting each twin pair as one delivery. ($p = 0.05$ if $\chi^2 \cong 3.84$).

APPENDIX 3.2. Treatment and Neonatal Death: Life table analysis

Completed weeks gestation	Supplement vs controls	Supplement vs complement	Complement vs controls	Supplement vs complement and controls combined
19	0.00	0.00	0.00	0.00
20	0.49	0.55	0.00	0.00
21	0.49	0.55	0.00	1.61
22	0.49	0.55	0.00	1.61
23	0.49	0.55	0.00	1.61
24	0.49	0.00	0.00	1.61
25	2.19	0.92	0.00	0.39
26	1.08	0.59	0.01	3.08
27	1.72	1.13	0.01	1.46
28	2.44	1.76	0.01	2.48
29	3.22	0.90	0.41	3.67
30	3.22	0.90	0.41	3.05
31	3.22	0.90	0.41	3.05
32	3.22	0.44	0.90	3.05
33	2.06	0.44	0.31	2.32
34	2.06	0.44	0.31	1.75
35	2.76	0.81	0.31	1.75
36 weeks and over	2.76	0.81	0.31	2.63

x^2 values for comparisons of cumulative neonatal death rates among life tables of treatment groups, including all participants at each stage of gestation, with twins counted as 2 births.
($p \leqslant 0.05$ if $x^2 \cong 3.84$)

APPENDIX 3.3. Individual Data on Neonatal Death: Selected characteristics of mothers, pregnancies, and their infants, for each neonatal death by treatment group among participants active to delivery

Case #	Average wt gain (lbs/wk)	# cigs/day at registration	Parity	Past perinatal loss (n)	Past low birthweight (n)	# days on study	Gestation at delivery (days)	Birthweight (gms)	Age at expiration (days)	Autopsy	Diagnosis
Treatment group Supplement											
1	1.03	30	2	0	0	53	143	567 } twins	1	No	Prematurity, RDS*, ecchymosis.
2								624		No	Prematurity, RDS, ecchymosis.
3	1.22	30	2	0	2	113	182	1048	3	No	Prematurity, RDS.
4	0.45	0	1	0	0	63	181	624	1	Yes	Prematurity, prem. rupture of membranes
5	−0.63	0	0	—	—	40	205	907	3	Yes	Prematurity, prolapsed cord, RDS.
6	0.35	10	0	—	—	39	194	1800	2	No	Prematurity, RDS.
7	0.69	10	1	1	1	34	197	unknown	1	No	Prematurity, died immediately.
8	−0.71	0	1	0	0	92	178	1021	3	Yes	Prematurity, RDS.
9	0.85	5	0	—	—	52	183	964	3	No	Prematurity, RDS, prem. rupture of membrane.
10	0.36	6	4	0	3	58	245	1432	5	Yes	Prematurity, GI perforation.
Mean	0.29 ± 0.57	10.1 ± 11.3	1.2 ± 1.2		1.0 ± 1.2	60 ± 25	190 ± 26	999 ± 381			

APPENDIX 3.3. (continued)

APPENDIX 3.3. (continued)

Case #	Average wt gain (lbs/w)	# cigs/day at registration	Past perinatal loss (n)	Past low birthweight (n)	# days on study	Gestation at delivery (days)	Birthweight (gms)	Age at expiration (days)	Autopsy	Diagnosis
Complement										
1	0.92	10	2	0	100	174	666	1	No	Prematurity, RDS.
2	1.02	8	0	—	29	184	798 } twins	1	No	Prematurity, RDS.
3							1026		No	Prematurity, RDS.
4	1.19	10	0	—	124	204	1120 (twin)	1	No	Prematurity; twin sib survived.
5	1.32	7	0	—	47	226	3175	4	Transferred	Congenital heart disease (cyanotic), sepsis.
6	0.61	0	1	2	109	209	1114	3	No	Prematurity, RDS, dissem. intravascular coagulopathy
Mean	1.01±0.24	7.0±3.7	1.2±1.6	1.0±1.0	82±37	199±18	1317±848			
Control										
1	0.53	20	1	1	36	235	2381	1	Yes	Congenital pneumonia.
2	−4.79	0	0	2	15	186	1048	1	Yes	Prematurity, atelectasis, subarachnoid hemorrhage
3	0.29	0	0	0	109	184	1729	8	No	Prolonged rupture of membranes, amnionitis
Mean	−1.32±2.45	6.7±9.4	2.7±1.7	1.0±0.8	53±40	202±24	1719±544			

*Respiratory Distress Syndrome

APPENDIX 3.4. Newborn Dimensions, Weight Gain, Diet, and Smoking

Newborn dimension	Weight gain		Averaged diet recalls		Cigarettes/day at registration
	Early	Average	Calories	Protein	
Birthweight					
Supplement	0.19**	0.33***	0.05	0.02	−0.05
Complement	0.13	0.15*	0.12	0.13	−0.12
Control	0.24***	0.26***	0.02	0.02	−0.24***
All	0.19***	0.25***	0.06	0.04	−0.13***
Length					
Supplement	0.14*	0.22*	−0.01	0.01	−0.08
Complement	0.06	0.08	−0.02	−0.04	−0.10
Control	0.07	0.13*	−0.06	−0.06	−0.19**
All	0.06	0.15***	−0.03	−0.03	−0.12**
Ponderal index (wt/ht^2)					
Supplement	0.14	0.22**	0.04	0.02	−0.04
Complement	0.08	0.13*	0.19**	0.22***	−0.08
Control	0.11	0.18**	−0.02	0.01	−0.11
All	0.11**	0.18***	0.07	0.07	−0.08*
Head circumference					
Supplement	0.15*	0.21**	0.04	0.04	−0.09
Complement	0.01	0.13	0.19**	0.23***	−0.16
Control	0.04	0.15*	−0.03	−0.02	−0.14*
All	0.07	0.17***	0.07	0.08*	−0.12**
Duration of gestation					
Supplement	0.02	0.16**			
Complement	0.01	−0.05			
Control	0.02	0.00			
All	0.01	0.05			

APPENDIX 3.4 (continued)

APPENDIX 3.4 (continued)

Newborn dimension	Weight gain		Averaged diet recalls		Cigarettes/day at registration
	Early	Average	Calories	Protein	
Arm girth					
Supplement	0.05	0.20**	−0.02	−0.03	−0.01
Complement	0.05	0.10	0.13	0.18**	−0.11
Control	0.09	0.12	0.06	0.07	−0.16*
All	0.07	0.14***	0.06	0.06	−0.09*
Triceps skinfold					
Supplement	0.11	0.18**	−0.09	−0.01	−0.04
Complement	0.07	0.09	−0.08	−0.03	−0.14*
Control	0.06	0.18*	−0.18**	−0.10	−0.17**
All	0.08*	0.18***	−0.11**	−0.04	−0.12**
Subscapular skinfold					
Supplement	0.16*	0.25***	0.00	0.07	−0.08
Complement	0.03	0.11	0.10	0.14*	−0.09
Control	0.04	0.09	−0.11	−0.08	−0.17**
All	0.08	0.15***	0.00	0.03	−0.11**
Placental weight					
Supplement	0.24**	0.28***	−0.03	−0.05	0.02
Complement	0.04	0.14	0.05	0.04	0.00
Control	0.14	0.19**	−0.05	−0.04	0.07
All	0.14***	0.21***	0.00	0.00	0.03

Selected newborn dimensions correlated, within treatment groups, with weight gain, diet intake, and smoking among 768 liveborn singletons.
  *$p < 0.05$
  **$p < 0.01$
  ***$p < 0.001$

APPENDIX 3.5a. Birthweight and Treatment: Multiple regression analysis

Step in multiple regression analysis	Variable	Regression coefficient (B); gm	F value for regression coefficient	Change in R^2 at entry	F value for change in R^2
1	Parity (n)	63.7	14.38	0.002	1.52
2	Past low bw infants (n)	−209.0	32.67	0.050	40.25
3	Cigarettes/d, at registration (n)	−7.5	8.01	0.011	8.96
4	Weight at conception (lbs)	−1.6	0.33	0.017	14.33
5	Stage gestation at registration (d)	−1.1	5.09	0.001	0.64
6	Weight at registration (lbs)	8.6	11.53	0.014	11.72
7	[a]Initial diet recall not completed = 1, others = 0	−173.2	2.94	0.005	4.0
8	Protein intake, 24 hr prior to registration (gm)	0.2	0.16	0.000	0.25
9	Supplement = 1, others = 0	−13.9	0.09	0.001	1.02
10	Complement = 1, others = 0	56.1	1.43	0.002	1.43
	Constant	2,255.2			

Stepwise multiple regression analysis with birthweight (gm) as dependent variable, and several variables including group as independent variables (n = 759; 8 cases with birthweight deviant for gestation omitted).

[a]n = 33.

R = Multiple correlation.

Change in R^2 at entry is the change in variance associated with variable entered at that step in analysis controlling for all variables previously entered. F at entry = F value associated with the variable, controlling for all variables previously entered. $p = 0.05$, $F = 3.84$; $p = 0.01$, $F = 6.63$; $p = 0.001$, $F = 10.83$.

APPENDIX 3.5b. Birthweight and Treatment: Multiple regression analysis

Step in multiple regression analysis	Variable	Regression coefficient (B); gm	F value for regression coefficient	Change in R^2 at entry	F value for change in R^2
1	Parity (n)	37.1	7.29	0.002	1.52
2	Past low bw infants (n)	−123.0	16.67	0.050	40.25
3	Cigarettes/d, at registration (n)	−7.2	11.23	0.011	8.96
4	Weight at conception (lbs)	−5.4	5.81	0.017	14.33
5	Stage gestation at registration (d)	−1.2	8.83	0.001	0.64
6	Weight at registration (lbs)	9.8	22.82	0.014	11.72
7	[a]Initial diet recall not completed = 1, others = 0	52.1	0.39	0.005	4.0
8	Protein intake, 24 hr prior to registration (gm)	−0.15	0.11	0.000	0.25
9	Gestation at delivery (d)	14.5	379.16	0.304	381.97
10	Supplement = 1, others = 0	−39.0	1.02	0.001	1.26
11	Complement = 1, others = 0	−2.5	0.00	0.000	0.00
	Constant	−1,330.5			

Stepwise multiple regression analysis with birthweight (gm) as dependent variable, and several variables including group as independent variables (n = 759; 8 cases with birthweight deviant for gestation omitted).

[a]n = 33

R = Multiple correlation

Change in R^2 at entry is the change in variance associated with variable entered at that step in analysis controlling for all variables previously entered. F at entry = F value associated with the variable, controlling for all variables previously entered. p = 0.05, F = 3.84; p = 0.01, F = 6.63; p = 0.001, F = 10.83.

APPENDIX 3.5c. Birthweight and Treatment: Multiple regression analysis

Step in multiple regression analysis	Variable	Regression coefficient (B); gm	F value for regression coefficient	Change in R^2 at entry	F value for change in R^2
1	Parity (n)	57.3	5.80	0.002	1.52
2	Past low bw infants (n)	−117.1	3.55	0.050	40.25
3	Cigarettes/d, at registration (n)	−17.4	11.84	0.011	8.96
4	Weight at conception (lbs)	−1.4	0.25	0.017	14.33
5	Stage gestation at registration (d)	−1.1	5.05	0.001	0.64
6	Weight at registration (lbs)	8.5	11.32	0.014	11.72
7	[a] Initial diet recall not completed = 1, others = 0				
8	Protein intake, 24 hr prior to registration (gm)	−164.1	2.60	0.005	4.0
		0.28	0.26	0.000	0.25
9	Supplement = 1, others = 0	−62.8	1.02	0.001	1.02
10	Complement = 1, others = 0	31.8	0.27	0.002	1.43
11	1 × 9	11.5	0.08	0.000	0.13
12	2 × 9	−160.6	3.21	0.001	0.97
13	1 × 10	15.3	0.15	0.000	0.01
14	2 × 10	−111.9	1.65	0.001	1.05
15	3 × 9	17.3	6.84	0.006	4.97
16	3 × 10	9.3	1.88	0.002	1.88
	Constant	2,257.7			

Stepwise multiple regression analysis with birthweight (gm) as dependent variable, and several variables including treatment group as independent variables (n = 759; 8 cases with birthweight deviant for gestation omitted).

[a] n = 33.

R = Multiple correlation

Change in R^2 at entry is the change in variance associated with variable entered at that step in analysis controlling for all variables previously entered. F at entry = F value associated with the variable, controlling for all variables previously entered. $p = 0.05$, $F = 3.84$; $p = 0.01$, $F = 6.63$; $p = 0.001$, $F = 10.83$.

APPENDIX 3.5d. Birthweight and Treatment: Multiple regression analysis

Step in multiple regression analysis	Variable	Regression coefficient (B); gm	F value for regression coefficient	Change in R^2 at entry	F value for change in R^2
1	Parity (n)	41.2	4.47	0.002	1.52
2	Past low bw infants (n)	−98.8	3.78	0.050	40.25
3	Cigarettes/d, at registration (n)				
4	Weight at conception (lbs)	−11.4	7.55	0.011	8.96
5	Stage gestation at registration (d)	−5.3	5.66	0.017	14.33
6	Weight at registration (lbs)	−1.2	8.84	0.001	0.64
7	[a]Initial diet recall not completed = 1, others = 0	9.9	22.76	0.014	11.72
8	Protein intake, 24 hr prior to registration (gm)	60.9	0.53	0.005	4.0
9	Gestation at delivery (d)	−0.07	0.02	0.000	0.25
10	Supplement = 1, others = 0	14.5	368.30		381.97
11	Complement = 1, others = 0	−69.3	1.86		1.26
12	1 × 10	12.6	0.06		0.00
13	2 × 10	4.7	0.02	0.000	0.55
14	1 × 11	−14.7	0.04	0.000	0.17
15	2 × 11	−18.0	0.30	0.001	0.91
16	3 × 10	−49.5	0.48	0.000	0.32
17	3 × 11	7.3	1.80	0.001	1.38
	Constant	3.6	0.43	0.000	0.43
		−1,333.6			

Stepwise multiple regression analysis with birthweight (gm) as dependent variable, and several variables including treatment group as independent variables (n = 759; 8 cases with birthweight deviant for gestation omitted).
[a] n = 33.
R = Multiple correlation.
Change in R^2 at entry is the change in variance associated with variable entered at that step in analysis controlling for all variables previously entered. F at entry = F value associated with the variable, controlling for all variables previously entered. p = 0.05, F = 3.84; p = 0.01, F = 6.63; p = 0.001, F = 10.83.

APPENDIX 3.5e. Birthweight and Diet Intake: Multiple regression analysis

Step in multiple regression analysis	Variable	Regression coefficient (B); gm	F value for regression coefficient	Change in R^2 at entry	F value for change in R^2
1	Parity (n)	−39.8	8.43	0.002	1.52
2	Past low bw infants (n)	−120.1	16.04	0.050	40.25
3	Cigarettes/d, at registration (n)	−7.8	13.15	0.011	8.96
4	Weight at conception (lbs)	−5.8	6.74	0.017	14.33
5	Stage gestation at registration (d)	−1.3	10.04	0.001	0.64
6	Weight at registration (lbs)	10.3	25.03	0.014	11.72
7	[a]Initial diet recall not completed = 1, others = 0	51.2	0.37	0.005	4.0
8	Protein intake, 24 hr prior to registration (gm)	−0.4	0.84	0.000	0.25
9	[b]No data, diet intake during study = 1, others = 0	78.9	0.97	0.007	6.13
10	Average calories/day during study	0.11	8.14	0.005	4.46
11	Average protein/day during study (gm)	−1.59	3.68	0.001	1.05
12	Gestation at delivery (d)	14.5	375.65	0.296	375.65
	Constant	−1,416.8			

Stepwise multiple regression analysis with birthweight (gm) as dependent variable, and several independent variables, including calorie and protein intake reported during study (n = 759; 8 cases with birthweight deviant for gestation omitted).

[a]n = 33.
[b]n = 54.

R = multiple correlation.

Change in R^2 at entry is the change in variance associated with variable entered at that step in analysis controlling for all variables previously entered. F at entry = F value associated with the variable, controlling for all variables previously entered. $p = 0.05$, $F = 3.84$; $p = 0.01$, $F = 6.63$; $p = 0.001$, $F = 10.83$.

APPENDIX 4.1. Psychological Indices at Age One

	Bayley scales		Object permanence	Play observation			Habituation	Dishabituation
	Mental	Motor		Sophistication	Number of episodes	Mean duration		
Bayley scales								
Mental		0.51***	0.45***	0.60***	0.18***	−0.06	−0.04	0.02
Motor	0.51***		0.37***	0.29***	0.21***	0.00	−0.07	0.11*
Object permanence	0.45***	0.37***		0.32***	0.22***	−0.15**	0.06	−0.03
Play observation								
Sophistication	0.60***	0.29***	0.33***		0.08	−0.10	−0.04	−0.02
No. of episodes	0.18***	0.21***	0.22***	0.08		−0.32***	−0.02	0.03
Mean duration	−0.06	0.00	−0.15**	−0.20	−0.32***		0.07	0.04
Habituation	−0.04	−0.07	0.06	−0.04	−0.02	0.07		−0.34***
Dishabituation	0.02	0.11*	−0.03	−0.02	0.03	0.04	−0.34***	
Somatic measures at age one								
Weight	0.10**	0.15***	−0.02	0.12*	0.00	−0.04	−0.08	0.07
Height	0.26***	0.26***	0.15***	0.16**	0.15**	−0.11*	−0.08	0.07
Head circumference	0.24***	0.18***	0.14**	0.24***	0.08	−0.03	0.01	0.04
Wt/Ht^2	−0.06	0.00	−0.13**	−0.10	−0.10	0.04	0.02	0.03
Arm circumferences	0.05	0.04	0.01	0.14**	−0.06	−0.07	−0.12*	0.03
Skinfold thickness								
Triceps	0.04	0.00	0.05	0.04	0.07	−0.05	−0.01	0.01
Subscapular	0.03	0.04	−0.07	0.02	0.00	0.02	−0.07	0.10
Birthweight	0.24***	0.27***	0.07	0.21***	0.10*	−0.05	−0.07	0.10
Duration of gestation	0.27***	0.25***	0.06	0.16**	0.12*	0.01	−0.08	0.00

Intercorrelations, and correlations with current and prior indices of growth. (All measures at age one standardized for chronologic age and sex.)
*p < 0.05
**p < 0.01
***p < 0.001

APPENDIX 4.2. Correlations of Somatic and Psychological Indices

Outcome variable	Duration of gestation < 37 weeks					
	Stage of gestation at recruitment					
	< 15 weeks			≥ 15 weeks		
	Supp	Comp	Cont	Supp	Comp	Cont
Weight	−0.23	−0.19	0.58*	0.08	−0.17	0.07
Height	−0.13	0.12	0.00	0.18	−0.23*	0.03
Head circumference	0.11	−0.15	0.05	−0.03	−0.15	0.16
Arm girth	−0.22	−0.26	0.44**	0.08	−0.14	0.04
Triceps skinfold	0.04	−0.37*	0.32*	0.06	−0.04	−0.02
Subscapular skinfold	−0.04	−0.44**	0.46**	0.04	0.03	−0.06
Bayley scales:						
Mental	0.14	0.03	−0.15	0.12	−0.24*	0.09
Motor	−0.04	−0.02	0.05	−0.05	−0.10	0.14
Play observation:						
Sophistication (Hunt-Uzgiris scale)	0.13	−0.23	0.09	0.10	−0.29*	0.16
New episodes	0.30	−0.41*	0.15	0.15	−0.06	0.09
Mean duration of episodes	−0.22	0.16	0.03	−0.05	−0.12	0.14
Object permanence Escalona-Corman scale	0.10	0.05	−0.13	0.16	−0.11	−0.07
Visual habituation:						
Habituation	−0.27	0.47*	−0.27	0.07	−0.14	0.05
Dishabituation	0.12	−0.21	0.12	0.23	−0.08	−0.14
Maximum No.	10	15	17	27	21	38

Correlations of somatic and psychological indices at age one with treatment group assignment within strata defined by a) gestation at entry into the study, b) gestation at delivery. (Each correlation coefficient is for the contrast of the treatment group in question versus the other two groups.)

*$p < 0.05$
**$p < 0.01$

APPENDIX 4.2 (continued)

APPENDIX 4.2 (continued)

Outcome variable	Duration of gestation					
	< 37 weeks			≥ 37 weeks		
	Total			Stage of gestation at recruitment < 15 weeks		
	Supp	Comp	Cont	Supp	Comp	Cont
Weight	0.00	−0.18*	0.17	0.01	0.08	−0.09
Height	0.08	−0.11	0.02	0.01	0.00	−0.01
Head circumference	0.01	−0.14	0.12	−0.03	0.04	−0.01
Arm girth	−0.02	−0.18*	0.17	0.05	0.11	−0.15*
Triceps skinfold	0.05	−0.16	0.10	−0.07	0.04	0.03
Subscapular skinfold	0.01	−0.16	0.14	−0.04	0.09	−0.05
Bayley scales:						
Mental	0.13	−0.15	0.02	0.03	−0.10	0.07
Motor	−0.05	−0.06	0.10	0.04	−0.07	0.03
Play observation:						
Sophistication (Hunt-Uzgiris scale)	0.10	−0.27*	0.14	−0.02	0.00	0.02
New episodes	0.20	−0.19	−0.01	−0.12	0.19*	−0.07
Mean duration of episodes	−0.09	−0.05	0.12	0.22*	−0.15	−0.07
Object permanence:						
Escalona-Corman scale	0.15	−0.06	−0.08	0.02	−0.01	−0.01
Visual habituation:						
Habituation	−0.03	0.07	−0.04	−0.15	0.08	0.07
Dishabituation	0.19	−0.14	−0.04	0.02	0.12	−0.14
Maximum No.	37	36	55	58	67	75

	Duration of gestation					
	≥ 37 weeks					
	Stage of gestation at recruitment					
	≥ 15 weeks			Total		
	Supp	Comp	Cont	Supp	Comp	Cont
	0.06	0.02	−0.09	0.05	0.04	−0.09*
	0.02	0.00	−0.01	0.02	0.00	−0.02
	0.05	−0.03	−0.02	0.02	−0.01	−0.02
	0.04	−0.03	−0.02	0.05	0.02	−0.07
	0.01	0.00	−0.01	−0.03	0.01	0.01
	0.14*	−0.07	−0.08	0.07	−0.01	−0.06
	−0.09	0.01	0.08	−0.04	−0.04	0.08
	−0.01	0.05	−0.04	0.00	0.00	0.00
	−0.01	−0.03	0.04	−0.02	−0.02	0.03
	−0.05	0.08	−0.03	−0.08	0.12*	−0.05
	0.12	−0.09	−0.04	0.16**	−0.11*	−0.05
	−0.07	−0.05	0.13	−0.04	−0.04	0.08
	−0.16*	0.16*	0.01	−0.16**	0.12*	0.03
	0.17*	−0.10	−0.07	0.11	−0.01	−0.10
	106	105	89	164	172	164

APPENDIX 4.3. Somatic Indices at Age One

	Weight				Height			
	Supp	Comp	Cont	Total	Supp	Comp	Cont	Total
Maternal attributes:								
Past low bw (n)[a]	0.03	−0.27**	−0.19*	−0.16**	−0.12	−0.22*	−0.13*	−0.16**
Married=1, others=0	0.00	0.20**	0.07	0.09*				
Family income								
On welfare=1, others=0	−0.09	−0.16	−0.13	−0.12**	−0.08	−0.12	−0.16*	−0.12**
Occup status, mat GF								
At conception								
Weight	0.18	0.09	0.17*	0.12**	0.23***	0.19**	0.27***	0.21***
Height	0.09	0.09	0.09	0.12**	0.15*	0.24***	0.28***	0.25***
At registration								
Weight	0.14	0.06	0.19**	0.13**	0.20**	0.12	0.26***	0.20***
Arm girth								
No. cigarettes/day								
No. gms protein/24 hr	0.09	0.06	0.18**	0.11**				
Low wt gain = 1 others=0					−0.10	−0.03	−0.17**	−0.11**
During study								
Early wt gain	0.13	0.06	0.20**	0.13**	0.15	0.05	0.14	0.12**
Average wt gain	0.18*	0.18*	0.28***	0.22***	0.26***	0.21**	0.25***	0.24***
1st recall, post regis: bevg protein								
Health aide's questionnaire:								
No. cans/day:								
past 24 hr								
past week								
Can count					0.15	0.19*		−0.17**
Smoking up to delivery=1, others=0					−0.13	−0.19**	−0.06	−0.12**
Attributes at birth:								
Duration of gestation	0.16*	0.16*	−0.02	0.10*	0.12	0.21**	0.26***	0.19***
Birthweight	0.25***	0.29***	0.33***	0.29***	0.33***	0.36***	0.37***	0.35***
Length of infant	0.21**	0.27***	0.23**	0.23***	0.32***	0.38***	0.22**	0.30***
Head circumference of infant	0.22**	0.25***	0.23***	0.23***	0.25***	0.29***	0.31***	0.28***
Arm girth of infant	0.16*	0.09	0.25***	0.17***	0.22**	0.17*	0.24***	0.21***
Triceps skinfold of infant	0.03	0.15*	0.15*	0.11**	0.13	0.12	0.09	0.11**
Subscapular skinfold of infant					0.02	0.20**	0.05	0.09*
Placental wt	0.21*	0.16*	0.17*	0.18***	0.23**	0.12	0.17*	0.18***

	Head circumference				Arm girth			
	Supp	Comp	Cont	Total	Supp	Comp	Cont	Total
	−0.26*	−0.15	−0.20*	−0.20***				
					−0.03	0.20**	0.09	0.08
	0.00	0.12	0.21**	0.11*				
	−0.06	−0.18**	0.19**	−0.15***				
	0.12	0.21***	0.15*	0.17***				
	0.14	0.17*	0.15*	0.15***				
	0.18**	0.17*	0.16*	0.17***				
	0.10	0.09	0.16*	0.12**				
	−0.18*	−0.04	−0.17*	−0.13**				
	0.15*	0.15*	0.26***	0.19***	0.05	0.07	0.18**	0.10*
	0.02	0.23**		0.07				
	0.15*	0.20**	0.08	0.14***				
	0.38***	0.43***	0.33***	0.37***	0.20**	0.21**	0.17*	0.19***
	0.29***	0.36***	0.16*	0.26***	0.17*	0.31***	0.10	0.18***
	0.46***	0.53***	0.47***	0.48***				
	0.24***	0.23**	0.15*	0.20***				
	0.15*	0.17*	0.16*	0.16***				
	0.23**	0.24**	0.19*	0.22***	0.20*	0.11	0.08	0.15**

APPENDIX 4.3 (continued)

APPENDIX 4.3. Somatic Indices at Age One

	Triceps skinfold				Subscapular skinfold			
	Supp	Comp	Cont	Total	Supp	Comp	Cont	Total
Maternal attributes:								
Past low bw (n)[a]								
Married = 1, others = 0								
Family income	0.11	0.21**	−0.02	0.11*				
On welfare = 1, others = 0								
Occup status, mat GF	0.05	−0.17	−0.26**	−0.14**				
At conception:								
Weight	0.02	0.20**	0.01	0.08				
Height	0.01	0.20**	0.02	0.08*				
At registration:								
Weight	0.02	0.22**	−0.05	0.06				
Arm girth								
No. cigarettes/day	0.01	0.08	−0.15*	−0.11**				
No. gms protein/24 hr								
Low wt gain = 1 others = 0					−0.13	−0.15*	−0.04	−0.11**
During study								
Early wt gain								
Average wt gain					0.06	0.06	0.18**	0.10*
1st recall, post regis: bevg protein								
Health aide's questionnaire:								
No. cans/day:								
past 24 hr					−0.08	0.21**		0.07
past week					−0.03	0.20**		0.09
Can count								
Smoking up to delivery = 1, others = 0								
Attributes at birth:								
Duration of gestation					0.08	0.07	−0.19**	−0.02
Birthweight	0.08	0.28***	0.09	0.15***	0.16*	0.17*	0.08	0.13***
Length of infant								
Head circumference of infant	0.00	0.24***	0.15*	0.13**	0.13	0.13	0.10	0.12**
Arm girth of infant	0.07	0.22**	0.07	0.11**				
Triceps skinfold of infant								
Subscapular skinfold of infant	−0.02	0.31***	0.07	0.12**	0.15*	0.19*	0.03	0.12**
Placental wt								

Relationship to maternal and prior infant characteristics, within treatment groups, and for total population. Set of four correlations (within three treatment groups, and total) shown only if at least one significant at p < 0.01 level.

[a]Multiparae only. *p < 0.05; **p < 0.01; ***p < 0.001.

APPENDIX 4.4. Psychological Indices at Age One

	Bayley scales							
	Mental				Motor			
	Supp	Comp	Cont	Total	Supp	Comp	Cont	Total
Maternal attributes:								
Past low bw (n)[a]	−0.12	−0.21*	−0.14	−0.16**	−0.22*	−0.30**	−0.13	−0.21***
Past stillbirth (n)[a]					0.24*	0.27**	0.01	0.15**
Mother's education (years)	0.10	0.19**	0.03	0.10*	0.14*	0.20**	0.02	0.11**
On welfare=1, others=0	−0.09	−0.19**	−0.04	−0.11**	−0.12	−0.20**	−0.12	−0.14**
Students=1, others=0	−0.11	0.05	0.24***	0.07				
Foreign born=1, others=0	−0.19**	−0.04	0.00	−0.07				
At conception:								
Height								
Ponderal Index (wt/ht^2)								
At registration:								
Stage of gestation	−0.20**	−0.08	−0.08	−0.11**	−0.13	−0.08	−0.10	−0.10**
Arm girth								
Subscapular skinfold								
Low wt gain=1, others=0								

APPENDIX 4.4 (continued)

APPENDIX 4.4 (continued)

	Bayley scales							
	Mental				Motor			
	Supp	Comp	Cont	Total	Supp	Comp	Cont	Total
During study:								
Avg calories/day	0.00	0.20**	0.07	0.09*				
Avg protein/day								
Calories, without beverage	0.02	0.19**	0.07	0.10*				
Protein, without beverage								
(Log) urine riboflavin								
No. cans/d, past wk	−0.20**	0.00		−0.09				
Began smoking=1, nonsmokers=0								
Infant attributes:								
Duration of gestation	0.25***	0.29***	0.29***	0.27***	0.25***	0.34***	0.17*	0.25***
Birthweight	0.18*	0.28***	0.27***	0.24***	0.23**	0.32***	0.28***	0.27***
Length at birth					0.12	0.24**	0.07	0.14**
Head circumference at birth	0.17*	0.36***	0.22**	0.25***	0.15*	0.22**	0.18*	0.18***
Arm girth at birth	0.23**	0.22**	0.34***	0.26***	0.14	0.13	0.29***	0.19***
At one year:								
Weight					0.08	0.26***	0.13	0.15***
Height	0.28***	0.24***	0.26***	0.26***	0.26***	0.25***	0.26***	0.26***
Head circumference	0.13	0.37***	0.22**	0.24***	0.09	0.35***	0.11	0.18***
Arm girth								
Triceps skinfold								

APPENDIX 4.4 (continued)

	Play observation											
	Sophistication (Uzgiris-Hunt scale)				No. of episodes				Mean duration			
	Supp	Comp	Cont	Total	Supp	Comp	Cont	Total	Supp	Comp	Cont	Total
Maternal attributes:												
Past low bw (n)[a]	−0.35**	−0.20	−0.30*	−0.28***					0.00	−0.04	0.32**	0.06
Past stillbirth (n)[a]												
Mother's education (years)												
On welfare = 1, others = 0												
Students = 1 others = 0												
Foreign born = 1, others = 0												
At conception:												
Height												
Ponderal Index (wt/ht²)	0.20*	−0.16	0.25**	0.10								
At registration:												
Stage of gestation	0.12	−0.07	0.27**	0.12*								
Arm girth												
Subscapular skinfold												
Low wt gain = 1, others = 0												

APPENDIX 4.4 (continued)

APPENDIX 4.4 (continued)

	Sophistication (Uzgiris-Hunt scale)				Play observation							
					No. of episodes				Mean duration			
	Supp	Comp	Cont	Total	Supp	Comp	Cont	Total	Supp	Comp	Cont	Total
During study:												
Avg calories/day					0.04	0.13	0.27**	0.14**				
Avg protein/day					0.06	0.14	0.28***	0.13*				
Calories, without beverage					0.05	0.10	0.27**	0.14**				
Protein, without beverage					0.09	0.13	0.28***	0.16**				
(Log) mean urine riboflavin												
No. cans/d, past wk												
Began smoking = 1, nonsmokers = 0												
Infant attributes:												
Duration of gestation	0.17	0.18	0.17*	0.16**	−0.03	0.25**	0.14	0.12*				
Birthweight	0.22*	0.23*	0.19*	0.21***								
Length at birth	0.17	0.28**	0.13	0.18***								
Head circumference at birth	0.33**	0.25**	0.20*	0.25***								
At one year:												
Weight	0.14	0.21*	0.14	0.16**	0.20*	0.11	0.14	0.15**				
Height												
Head circumference	0.26**	0.35***	0.12	0.24***								
Arm girth					0.16	0.26**	0.03	0.14**				
Triceps skinfold									−0.01	0.07	−0.21**	−0.05

APPENDIX 4.4 (continued)

Maternal attributes:	Object permanence (Escalona-Corman scale)				Habituation				Dishabituation			
	Supp	Comp	Cont	Total	Supp	Comp	Cont	Total	Supp	Comp	Cont	Total
Past low bw (n)[a]												
Past stillbirth (n)[a]												
Mother's education (years)												
On welfare = 1, others = 0												
Students = 1, others = 0												
Foreign born = 1, others = 0					−0.18*							
At conception:												
Height						−0.14	−0.17	−0.15**				
Ponderal Index (wt/ht²)												
At registration:												
Stage of gestation												
Arm girth												
Subscapular skinfold					−0.14	−0.29**	0.08	−0.10				
Low wt gain = 1, others = 0									0.08	0.09	−0.27**	−0.04

APPENDIX 4.4 (continued)

APPENDIX 4.4 (continued)

During study:	Object permanence (Escalona-Corman scale)				Habituation				Dishabituation			
	Supp	Comp	Cont	Total	Supp	Comp	Cont	Total	Supp	Comp	Cont	Total
Avg calories/day	0.05	0.27**	0.12	0.14**								
Avg protein/day												
Calories, without beverage	0.06	0.26**	0.12	0.15**								
Protein, without beverage	0.04	0.20*	0.03	0.09*								
(Log) urine riboflavin	−0.05	0.30***	—	0.11								
No. cans/d, past wk												
Began smoking = 1, nonsmokers = 0									−0.28*	0.31**	−0.05	0.05
Infant attributes:												
Duration of gestation												
Birthweight												
Length at birth												
Head circumference at birth	0.05	0.22**	−0.01	0.07								
Arm girth at birth												
At one year:												
Weight	0.27**	0.14	0.06	0.15***					0.00	−0.12	0.29**	0.07
Height	0.17*	0.15	0.12	0.14**								
Head circumference												
Arm girth	−0.24**	−0.01	−0.02	−0.12*	−0.24	0.05	−0.17	−0.12*				
Triceps skinfold												

Relationship to maternal and prior infant characteristics, within treatment groups, and for total population. Set of 4 correlations (within 3 treatment groups, and total) shown only if at least one significant at $p < 0.01$ level.

APPENDIX 4.5a. Bayley Mental Score and Treatment: Multiple regression analysis

Step in multiple regression analysis	Variable (units)	Regression coefficient (B)	F, regression coefficient	Change in R^2 at entry	F, change in R^2
1	Age at exam (days)	0.121	585.36	0.472	542.64
2	Sex (male = 1, female = 2)	0.202	0.17	0.000	0.03
3	Parity (n)	−0.294	1.85	0.002	2.00
4	Past low bw (n)	−0.413	0.83	0.006	7.46
5	Cigarettes/day at registration (n)	0.062	3.40	0.001	1.68
6	Weight at conception (lbs)	−0.009	0.06	0.002	1.81
7	Gestation at registration (d)	−0.015	5.67	0.005	6.18
8	Weight at registration (lbs)	0.025	0.58	0.001	0.73
9	[a]Protein intake at registration not available = 1, others = 0	2.259	3.22	0.001	0.34
10	Protein intake at registration (gm)	−0.0003	0.00		
11	Supplement vs others	−0.659	1.19	0.000	0.58
12	Complement vs others	−1.245	4.44	0.002	0.04
13	[b]Study diet intake not available = 1, others = 0	1.841	2.12	0.004	1.77
14	Calorie intake/day during study	0.0012	4.88		0.71
15	Protein intake/day during study (gm)	−0.011	0.85	0.000	4.77
16	Duration of gestation (d)	0.070	23.94	0.037	0.42
17	Birthweight (gm)	0.0017	8.11	0.006	47.24
					8.11

Stepwise multiple regression analysis with raw Bayley mental score as dependent variable, and several variables, including treatment group, as independent variables (n = 609). Constant = 30.942.
[a]n = 28, [b]n = 40. p = 0.05, F = 3.84; p = 0.01, F = 6.63; p = 0.001, F = 10.83.

APPENDIX 4.5b. Bayley Motor Score and Treatment: Multiple regression analysis

Step in multiple regression analysis	Variable (units)	Regression coefficient (B)	F, regression coefficient	Change in R^2 at entry	F, change in R^2
1	Age at exam (days)	0.051	353.12	0.344	323.20
2	Sex (male = 1, female = 2)	0.076	0.08	0.000	0.23
3	Parity (n)	−0.112	0.87	0.003	2.70
4	Past low bw (n)	−0.510	4.08	0.016	15.23
5	Cigarettes/d at registration (n)	0.017	0.81	0.000	0.09
6	Weight at conception (lbs)	−0.010	0.29	0.003	2.47
7	Gestation at registration (d)	−0.008	5.25	0.004	4.28
8	Weight at registration (lbs)	0.022	1.51	0.003	2.76
9	[a]Protein intake at registration not available = 1, others = 0	1.386	3.924	0.003	0.64
10	Protein intake at registration (gm)	0.004	0.82		1.91
11	Supplement vs others	−0.147	0.19	0.000	0.12
12	Complement vs others	−0.296	0.82	0.000	0.12
13	[b]Study diet intake not available = 1, others = 0	0.450	0.43	0.001	0.29
14	Calorie intake/day during study	0.004	1.38		0.43
15	Protein intake/day during study (gm)	−0.007	0.85	0.001	0.49
16	Duration of gestation (d)	0.030	14.32	0.036	36.52
17	Birthweight (gm)	0.001	13.78	0.013	13.78

Stepwise multiple regression analysis with raw Bayley motor score as dependent variable, and several variables, including treatment group, as independent variables (n = 619). Constant 15.214.
[a]n = 28, [b]n = 43. $p = 0.05$, $F = 3.84$; $p = 0.01$, $F = 6.63$; $p = 0.001$, $F = 10.83$.

APPENDIX 4.5c. Habituation and Treatment: Multiple regression analysis

Step in multiple regression analysis	Variable (units)	Regression coefficient (B)	F, regression coefficient	Change in R^2 at entry	F, change in in R^2
1	Age at exam (days)	−0.027	0.10	0.000	0.14
2	Sex (male = 1, female = 2)	−4.174	0.28	0.000	0.00
3	Parity (n)	−1.110	0.11	0.001	0.26
4	Past low bw (n)	7.573	0.98	0.007	2.75
5	Cigarettes/d at registration (n)	0.260	0.24	0.000	0.10
6	Weight at conception (lbs)	−0.867	2.18	0.008	3.07
7	Gestation at registration (d)	−0.134	1.65	0.004	1.58
8	Weight at registration (lbs)	0.267	0.23	0.001	0.59
9	[a]Protein intake at registration not available = 1, others = 0	−37.007	2.90	0.006	0.53
10	Protein intake at registration (gm)	−0.157	1.67		
11	Supplement vs others	−21.741	5.08	0.020	8.13
12	Complement vs others	12.880	1.82	0.003	1.25
13	[b]Study diet intake not available = 1, others = 0	−3.547	0.03	0.006	0.73
14	Calorie intake/day during study	−0.021	5.36		1.71
15	Protein intake/day during study (gm)	0.395	3.66	0.008	3.41
16	Duration of gestation (d)	−0.324	2.00	0.007	3.07
17	BW (gm)	−0.004	0.17	0.000	0.17

Stepwise multiple regression analysis with decline in duration of first fixation least squares slope as dependent variable, and several variables, including treatment group, as independent variables. (n = 398) Constant 156.195.
[a]n = 16, [b]n = 26. p = 0.05, F = 3.84; p = 0.01, F = 6.63; p = 0.001, F = 10.83.

APPENDIX 4.5d. Dishabituation and Treatment: Multiple regression analysis

Step in multiple regression analysis	Variable (units)	Regression coefficient (B); seconds	F, regression coefficient	Change in R^2 at entry	F, change in R^2
1	Age at exam (days)	0.003	0.05	0.000	0.01
2	Sex (male = 1, female = 2)	−0.143	0.02	0.003	1.08
3	Parity (n)	0.114	0.05	0.000	0.01
4	Past low bw (n)	−0.185	0.03	0.002	0.92
5	Cigarettes/d at registration (n)	−0.129	2.62	0.006	2.07
6	Weight at conception (lbs)	0.028	0.10	0.003	0.98
7	Gestation at registration (d)	0.001	0.00	0.000	0.06
8	Weight at registration (lbs)	0.019	0.05	0.001	0.28
9	[a]Protein intake at registration not available = 1, others = 0	1.522	0.20	0.001	0.17
10	Protein intake at registration (gm)	0.013	0.50		0.38
11	Supplement vs others	3.650	6.56	0.014	5.16
12	Complement vs others	−0.143	0.01	0.000	0.02
13	[b]Study diet intake not available = 1, others = 0	0.585	0.04		0.23
14	Calorie intake/day during study	0.002	1.93	0.001	0.11
15	Protein intake/day during study (gm)	−0.063	4.08	0.011	4.23
16	Duration of gestation (d)	−0.015	0.20	0.000	0.18
17	Birthweight (gm)	0.003	3.91	0.010	3.91

Stepwise multiple regression analysis with increased duration of first fixation of gaze in seconds with the presentation of a novel stimulus as dependent variable, and several variables, including treatment group, as independent variables (n = 375). Constant = 8.355, [a]n = 14, [b]n = 22. p = 0.05, F = 3.84; p = 0.01, F = 6.63; p = 0.001, F = 10.83.

APPENDIX 4.5e. Duration of Episodes of Play and Treatment: Multiple regression analysis

Step in multiple regression analysis	Variable (units)	Regression coefficient (B); seconds	F, regression coefficient	Change in R^2 at entry	F, change in R^2
1	Age at exam (days)	0.06	0.43	0.001	0.37
2	Sex (male = 1, female = 2)	14.44	2.57	0.005	1.93
3	Parity (n)	1.06	0.08	0.000	0.12
4	Past low bw (n)	2.90	0.11	0.000	0.02
5	Cigarettes/day at registration (n)	−0.70	1.17	0.001	0.41
6	Weight at conception (lbs)	−0.02	0.00	0.000	0.07
7	Gestation at registration (d)	−0.09	0.54	0.004	1.53
8	Weight at registration (lbs)	0.16	0.07	0.000	0.01
9	[a]Protein intake at registration, not available = 1, others = 0	−1.76	0.01	0.001	0.06
10	Protein intake at registration (gm)	−0.06	0.00		
11	Supplement vs others	23.09	4.12	0.014	6.17
12	Complement vs others	−14.81	1.82	0.003	1.19
13	[b]Study diet intake not available = 1, others = 0	18.34	0.69	0.012	4.31
14	Calorie intake/day during study	0.01	1.01		
15	Protein intake/day during study (gm)	−0.48	3.05	0.007	3.08
16	Duration of gestation (d)	0.20	0.60	0.001	0.22
17	Birthweight (gm)	−0.01	0.63	0.001	0.63

Stepwise multiple regression analysis with mean duration of discrete episodes of play, in seconds, as dependent variable and several variables, including treatment group, as independent variables (n = 427). Constant = 15.72.
[a]n = 21; [b]n = 32. p = 0.05, F = 3.84; p = 0.01, F = 6.63; p = 0.001, F = 10.83.

APPENDIX 5.1. Summary of Studies of Maternal Nutrition Intervention in Pregnancy

	Dutch Famine Study	Bogotá, Colombia	Guatemala/INCAP
STUDY OBJECTIVE	Impact of acute starvation during pregnancy on birthweight and subsequent development in 18-year-old men.	Effect of prenatal and postnatal nutritional supplementation on birthweight and child development.	Effect of prenatal and postnatal nutritional supplementation on birthweight, infant morbidity and mortality and child development.
RESEARCH DESIGN	Retrospective cohort study of records from maternity hospitals, vital records and military induction for cohort of all births to women exposed to acute famine during World War II. Control groups from comparable cohorts whose mothers were not exposed to famine. Records available of weekly food rations.	Prospective intervention study of offspring of women supplemented in third trimester and/or during lactation with food to meet recommended daily allowances; medical care provided. Random assignment with controls, but not blind.	Prospective pre- and postnatal supplementation study of pregnant and lactating women and of children up to age 7 years. Liquid supplements consumed in community center; medical care provided. Quasi experiment without random assignment.
DESCRIPTION OF POPULATION	Dutch cities under Nazi occupation, World War II. Famine exposed. n = 40,000 births well fed up to 1940; food rationing 1941–44. Near starvation, 1944–45, rehabilitation, 1945–46. Controls n = 80,000 not exposed to famine 1944–45.	n = 413 births. Urban slums. Pregnant women selected as having prior malnourished child. Estimated average daily intake: 1,600 calories, 35.5 gm protein.	n = 1,536 pregnancies. 4 rural villages. Estimated average daily intake for pregnant women: 1,400 calories, 45 gm protein.
DIETARY MODIFICATION	Gradual starvation over 6 months (external food supplies cut off 1944–45), then immediate restoration to high food intake.	Selected foods provided for entire family. Net increment for pregnant women was 133 calories and 20 gm protein daily.	Liquid supplements: 1) Fresco=low calorie, no protein; vitamin, mineral fortified. 2) Atole=proteins + calories; vitamin, mineral fortified. Ad libitum intake measured at individual level.

	Montreal	New York City	Taiwan
	Impact of prenatal dietary improvement program on birthweight and infant survival.	Impact of prenatal supplementation on birthweight and infant development.	Impact of prenatal and postnatal nutritional supplementation on birthweight, child development, and protein metabolism.
	Prospective study of patients entered through public prenatal clinic; supplement consisted of free extra foods based on dietary and clinical characterization; education and health care provided. Quasi experiment with retrospectively matched controls.	Prospective study of nutritional intervention of public prenatal clinic patients with follow-up of infants to 1 year of age; medical care provided. Randomized blind controlled trial.	Prospective study of liquid nutritional supplements or placebo provided to women for consumption in community health center. First child not treated; second child assigned randomly to treatment groups. Medical care provided.
	n = 1,213 white urban patients, 1,213 controls. Generally low income women.	n = 769 singleton births. Poor black urban women, identified as being "at risk" for low birthweight upon entrance to public prenatal clinic. Controls daily dietary intake at 2,065 calories, 79 gm protein.	n = 294 enrolled. 169 completed two pregnancies and consumed adequate supplements. Population from 14 rural villages (poor). Married women only with 1 prior male child. Basal daily dietary intake of women: 1,200 calories $<$ 40 gm protein.
	Free foods provided on "prescription basis" coupled with nutrition education; dietary histories taken regularly.	Liquid "Supplement": 470 calories plus 40 gm protein plus vitamins and minerals. Liquid "Complement": 322 calories plus 6 gm protein plus vitamins and mineral. Control: no calorie or protein supplement; routine vitamins and minerals.	Supplement A=800 calories; 40 gm protein. Supplement B = 80 calories; no protein. Control: no nutrition intervention.

APPENDIX 5.1 (continued)

APPENDIX 5.1 (continued)

	Dutch Famine Study	Bogotá, Colombia	Guatemala/INCAP
INCREASE IN BIRTH-WEIGHT FOLLOWING DIETARY IMPROVEMENT	Yes: 400 gm, maximum when diet improved in third trimester. Conversely, birthweight declined with third trimester famine exposure to a maximal mean decrement of 300 gm from prefamine level.	Yes: Average increment of 50 gm for all supplemented, 77 gm for those supplemented one trimester or more (not statistically significant). Data suggest increased birthweight associated with increased protein intake.	Yes: 28 gm per 10,000 supplemental calories consumed during pregnancy (based on 405 births). Data suggest increased birthweight associated with increased energy intake.
INFLUENCES OF GESTATIONAL AGE ON RESPONSE TO DIETARY CHANGE	Nutritional rehabilitation during third trimester was sufficient to restore mean birthweight to prefamine levels.	Last trimester or more showed effect.	No effect detected; birthweight increment depended on total calories ingested during pregnancy.
INFLUENCE OF SEX OF INFANT ON RESPONSE TO DIETARY CHANGE	At height of famine decrement in birthweight was greater for males than for females.	Increment in males (100 gm) greater than in females (12 gm).	None detected.
EFFECTS ON MOTHER	Maternal weight decrement at 10 days postnatal preceded decrease in birthweight. With alleviation of famine, maternal weight increased before birthweight did, and continued to increase as full feeding continued.	Greater maternal weight gain associated with supplementation.	Supplement intake associated with: increase in weight gain during pregnancy; in placental weight; in placental RNAase activity, and with shorter postpartum amenorrhea and shorter birth interval.

Montreal	New York City	Taiwan
Yes: 40 gm average increment. (Statistically significant.)	Yes: 41 gm reported with Complement (not statistically significant); 42 gm less with Supplement. Heavy smoking decreased birthweight. Supplement and Complement overcame the decrease in birthweight due to heavy smoking.	Yes: 349 gm advantage among females, and 799 among males (not statistically significant) for those consuming more than 50% of supplement A, compared to Supplement B and untreated controls.
No effect detected.	Birthweight not related to gestational age at which supplements were started.	Treatment before and during pregnancy; no effect detected.
Not analyzed.	None detected.	Differences not interpretable from published data.
Maternal weight gain not significantly increased by added dietary intake.	Maternal weight gain affected only women entering treatment early in pregnancy.	No effect of supplement A on maternal weight gain. Mothers on Supplement A excreted 1.2 gm N more than those on Supplement B, but consumed 4.8 gm N more.

APPENDIX 5.1 (continued)

APPENDIX 5.1 (continued)

	Dutch Famine Study	Bogotá, Colombia	Guatemala/INCAP
ADVERSE EFFECTS OBSERVED	Excess in the number of very early prematures and increased perinatal mortality, with starvation in the first trimester, could be due to the starvation or the rapid rehabilitation that followed.	None reported.	None detected.

ADDITIONAL OUTCOMES:

INFANT MORBIDITY AND MORTALITY	Prenatal starvation associated with increased infant mortality at least up to 90 days postpartum. First trimester famine exposure associated with excess CNS abnormalities; exposure in first half of pregnancy associated with excess obesity; exposure in last half of pregnancy and first months of life with reduction in obesity.	Supplementation associated with reduced perinatal mortality (not statistically significant). Later morbidity not yet analyzed.	No relationship between supplement consumption and duration of infant diarrhea; supplementation plus frequent medical care usage associated with decreased infant mortality (1,536 births).
BEHAVIORAL EFFECTS	None in young men with prenatal famine exposure.	More rapid habituation in supplemented 15-day-old infants.	Advanced psychomotor performance in supplemented (pre- and postnatal combined) infants and children to age four years.

Mexico	Montreal	New York City	Taiwan
None reported.	Birthweight of supplemented pregnancies with prior LBW infants lower than controls with similar history (not statistically significant).	Larger number of very premature deliveries, excess neonatal deaths, and depressed birthweight (among prematures only), with high protein Supplement, especially among those with prior LBW infants.	Not examined.
None reported.	None reported.	Not detected.	Not examined.
Supplemented infants "more active" throughout study.	Not studied.	Rapid habituation in Supplement group at 1 year; also increased duration of episodes of play. No changes in the usual developmental measures.	One significant effect among 22 subtests from the Bayley tests.

APPENDIX 6. Placental Biochemistry and Treatment[a]

	Supplement		
	< 37w	≥ 37w	Total
Placental weight (gm)	383.3 ± 102.2 (35)	447.0 ± 91.5 (143)	434.6 ± 96.3 (181)
Protein/gm (mg)	110.6 ± 117.3 (31)	109.4 ± 15.5 (112)	109.7 ± 15.9 (146)
DNA/gm (mg)	2.57 ± 0.37 (24)	2.62 ± 4.10 (109)	2.61 ± 0.40 (141)
RNA/gm (mg)	0.73 ± 0.26 (29)	0.71 ± 0.20 (109)	0.71 ± 0.22 (141)
Protein/DNA (mg/mg)	43.1 ± 6.1 (29)	42.3 ± 7.4 (109)	42.5 ± 7.1 (141)
RNA/DNA (mg/mg)	0.30 ± 0.10 (29)	0.27 ± 0.79 (109)	0.28 ± 0.08 (141)
RNase/gm (units/1000)	33.6 ± 8.4 (27)	31.8 ± 5.7 (100)	32.2 ± 6.4 (129)

[a]This appendix was developed with the help of Myron Winick, Pedro Rosso, and Mary Campbell Brown.

APPENDIX 7. Placental Histomorphometry and Treatment[a]

	Supplement		
	< 37w	≥ 37w	Total
Ratio, cytoplasmic/nuclear points:			
In deciduum	4.6 ± 2.0 (30)	6.0 ± 2.0 (109)	5.7 ± 2.1 (142)
In umbilicus	19.8 ± 7.6 (34)	21.9 ± 9.3 (134)	21.6 ± 9.1 (171)
In syncytium	14.6 ± 2.8 (34)	13.3 ± 3.2 (135)	13.5 ± 3.1 (172)
In villus	16.6 ±10.2 (34)	14.3 ± 8.0 (135)	14.8 ± 8.6 (172)
Villus, %:			
Collagen	28.1 ±13.8	29.5 ±12.4	29.3 ±12.6
Capillary	28.5 ±12.6	27.5 ±13.6	27.7 ±13.4
Other	38.8 ±16.0 (34)	38.0 ±14.8 (135)	38.2 ±15.1 (172)

[a]This appendix was developed with the help of Richard Naeye.

	Treatment group					
	Complement			Control		
	< 37w	≥ 37w	Total	< 37w	≥ 37w	Total
	388.6 ± 81.1 (32)	440.6 ± 88.2 (169)	432.3 ± 89.2 (201)	418.9 ± 108.9 (42)	429.9 ± 83.4 (152)	427.9 ± 84.7 (195)
	107.4 ± 14.3 (28)	111.8 ± 15.2 (122)	110.0 ± 15.1 (150)	106.9 ± 18.3 (32)	109.8 ± 15.2 (127)	109.2 ± 15.8 (160)
	2.58 ± 0.33 (26)	2.57 ± 0.40 (121)	2.57 ± 0.39 (147)	2.66 ± 0.40 (32)	2.62 ± 0.38 (125)	2.62 ± 0.38 (158)
	0.79 ± 0.30 (27)	0.75 ± 0.24 (121)	0.76 ± 0.25 (148)	0.78 ± 0.20 (32)	0.76 ± 0.24 (125)	0.76 ± 0.24 (158)
	41.8 ± 5.3 (26)	44.6 ± 8.7* (121)	44.1 ± 8.3* (147)	40.7 ± 7.2 (32)	42.7 ± 7.5 (124)	42.3 ± 7.4 (157)
	0.32 ± 0.11 (26)	0.29 ± 0.09 (121)	0.30 ± 0.09 (147)	0.30 ± 0.08 (32)	0.29 ± 0.08 (125)	0.29 ± 0.08 (158)
	34.1 ± 6.5 (23)	32.5 ± 5.8 (105)	32.7 ± 6.0 (128)	35.3 ± 7.6 (26)	32.5 ± 7.3 (115)	33.0 ± 7.4 (142)

Mean of placental weight and biochemical variables, by treatment group and duration of gestation (eight cases with birthweight deviant for gestation included in totals only). ( ) = n.
*$p < 0.05$ vs other two treatment groups combined.

	Treatment group					
	Complement			Control		
	< 37w	≥ 37w	Total	< 37w	≥ 37w	Total
	5.6 ± 2.4 (22)	6.1 ± 2.0 (114)	6.0 ± 2.1* (136)	4.6 ± 1.9 (33)	5.7 ± 1.9 (116)	5.4 ± 1.9 (142)
	19.6 ± 6.7 (26)	22.1 ± 9.8 (155)	21.7 ± 9.5 (181)	18.0 ± 6.2 (39)	21.6 ± 10.2 (144)	20.8 ± 9.6 (184)
	13.7 ± 3.5 (27)	13.4 ± 3.5 (159)	13.4 ± 3.5 (186)	14.4 ± 4.0 (39)	13.4 ± 3.2 (145)	13.6 ± 3.4 (185)
	12.2 ± 6.5 (27)	14.7 ± 8.1 (159)	14.4 ± 7.9 (186)	14.7 ± 8.4 (39)	16.3 ± 9.7* (145)	16.0 ± 9.4 (185)
	29.2 ± 16.0	29.8 ± 11.0	29.8 ± 11.9	32.5 ± 15.3	31.2 ± 11.4	31.4 ± 12.4
	26.9 ± 11.8	26.0 ± 12.4	26.1 ± 12.3	24.2 ± 12.1	23.9 ± 13.3*	24.0 ± 13.1*
	39.2 ± 17.9 (27)	38.9 ± 13.5 (159)	39.0 ± 14.2 (186)	38.7 ± 15.6 (39)	40.4 ± 15.6 (145)	40.0 ± 14.8 (185)

Means of placental histomorphometric variables, by treatment and duration of gestation (eight cases with birthweight deviant for gestation included in totals only).
( ) = n. *$p < 0.05$ vs other two treatment groups combined.

APPENDIX 8. Histopathology of Placenta[a]

	Treatment group			
	Supplement	Complement	Control	Total
Meconium histiocytes	11.4 (18)	12.7 (23)	11.1 (20)	11.8 (61)
Amnion nodosum	0.6 (1)	0.0	0.0	0.2 (1)
Chorioamnionitis, 1+	59.5 (94)	63.0 (114)	54.4 (98)	59.0 (306)
2+	6.3 (10)	3.3 (6)	4.4 (8)	4.6 (24)
3+	0.6 (1)	0.6 (1)	1.7 (3)	1.0 (5)
Total +	66.4 (105)	66.9 (121)	60.6 (109)	64.5 (335)
Chorionic Vessels:				
Myolysis	90.5 (143)	91.2 (165)	88.9 (160)	90.2 (468)
Thrombosis	0.6 (1)	2.2 (4)	4.4 (8)	2.5 (13)
Infarct	1.9 (3)	2.8 (5)	3.9 (7)	2.9 (15)
Villi:				
Inter-villus thrombosis	7.6 (12)	6.1 (11)	7.8 (14)	7.1 (37)
Inter-villus fibrin deposition	18.4 (29)	12.7 (23)	11.7 (21)	14.1 (73)
Stem villi pathology	27.8 (44)	23.2 (42)	22.2 (40)	24.3 (126)
Avascular villi	5.1 (8)	5.0 (9)	7.2 (13)	5.8 (30)
Focal edema	0.0	0.6 (1)	0.0	0.2 (1)
Micro infarcts	1.3 (2)	3.3 (6)	0.0	1.5 (8)
Excessive knotting	3.2 (5)	3.6 (6)	1.7 (3)	2.7 (14)
Hyperplasia	2.5 (4)	0.6 (1)	1.7 (3)	1.5 (8)
Villitis, viral type	13.9 (22)	17.1 (31)	13.9 (25)	15.0 (78)
Villitis, acute	5.1 (8)	2.8 (5)	2.2 (4)	3.3 (17)
Extramedullary hematopoiesis	0.1	1.1 (2)	0.6 (1)	0.6 (3)
Sickling	5.1 (8)	2.2 (4)	5.0 (9)	4.0 (21)
Decidua:				
Acute inflammation	48.3 (70)	41.4 (75)	44.3 (87)	44.7 (232)
Chronic inflammation	96.8 (153)	97.8 (177)	95.6 (172)	96.7 (502)
Atheroma	4.4 (7)	3.3 (6)	4.4 (8)	4.0 (21)
Umbilical Cord:				
Single artery	0.0	0.6 (1)	0.0	0.2 (1)
Funisitis, acute, 1+	22.8 (36)	24.9 (45)	24.4 (44)	24.1 (125)
2+	3.2 (5)	1.7 (3)	2.2 (4)	2.3 (12)
Total +	25.9 (41)	26.5 (48)	26.7 (48)	26.4 (137)
Funisitis, chronic	0.6 (1)	0.0	0.0	0.2 (1)
Premature, morphologically	26.6 (42)	35.4 (64)	32.8 (59)	31.8 (165)
Total number	158	181	180	519

[a]This appendix was developed with the help of William Blanc, Prem Chauhan, and Carlos Navarro.

Percentage abnormal findings, by treatment group, liveborn singletons.

( ) = number positive.

Definitions per Blanc et al [1978]; thanks to the Nestle Foundation for partial support for this analysis.

References

Barnes RH, Moore AU, Reid IM, Pond WG (1968): Effect of food deprivation on behavioral patterns. In Scrimshaw NS, Gordon JE (eds): "Malnutrition, Learning and Behavior." Cambridge: M.I.T. Press, pp 203–17.

Barnes RH, Moore AU, Pond WG (1970): Behavioral abnormalities in young adult pigs caused by malnutrition in early life. J Nutr 100: 149–55.

Belmont L, Marolla FA (1973): Birth order, family size and intelligence. Science 182:1096–101.

Belmont L, Stein ZA, Susser MW (1975): Comparison of associations of birth order with intelligence test score and height. Nature 255:54–6.

Benton AL (1940): Mental development of prematurely born children: a critical review of the literature. Am J Orthopsychiatry 10:719–46.

Bergner L, Susser MW (1970): Low birth weight and prenatal nutrition: an interpretative review. Pediatrics 46:946–66.

Birch HG, Gussow JD (1970): "Disadvantaged Children: Health, Nutrition and School Failure." New York: Grune and Stratton.

Birch HG, Richardson SA, Baird D, Horodin G, Illsley R (1973): "Mental Subnormality in the Community: A Clinical and Epidemiologic Study." Baltimore: Williams & Wilkins.

Blackwell RQ, Chow BF, Chinn KSK, Blackwell BN, Hsu SC (1973): Prospective maternal nutrition study in Taiwan: rationale, study design, feasibility, and preliminary findings. Nutr Rep Int 7(5): 517–32.

Blanc WA, Navarro C, Reinhardt MC (1978): The placentas in Abidjan. Helv Paediatr Acta 33 (Suppl 41):101–10.

Boelkins RC, Hegsted DM (1978): Consequences of early protein and energy malnutrition in monkeys. In Brozek J (ed): "Behavioral Consequences of Energy and Protein Deficits." Washington, DC: Proc Int Conf, PAHO.

Brazelton RB: "Fetal, Neonatal Behavioural Assessment Scale." Boston: Children's Hospital Medical Center, mimeographed, undated.

Brozek J, Coursin DB, Read MS (1977): Longitudinal studies on the effects of malnutrition, nutritional supplementation, and behavioral stimulation. PAHO Bulletin XI (3):237–49.

Chavez A, Martinez C (1975): Nutrition and development of children from poor rural areas. V. Nutrition and behavioural development. Nutr Rep Int 11:477–89.

Chow BF, Blackwell RQ, Blackwell B-N, Hou TY, Anilane JK, Sherwin RW (1968): Maternal nutrition and metabolism of the offspring: studies in rats and man. Am J Public Health 58:668–77.

Corman HH, Escalona SK (1969): Stages of sensorimotor development: a replication study. Merrill-Palmer Q 15:351–61.

Cravioto J, DeLicardie ER (1975): Environment and nutritional deprivation in children with learning disabilities. In Cruickshank WM, Hallahan DP (eds): "Perceptual and Learning Disabilities in Children: Volume 2, Research and Theory." Syracuse: Syracuse University Press, pp 3–102.

Crosby WM, Metcoff J, Costiloe JP, Mameesh M, Sandstead HH, Jacob RA, McClain PE, Jacobson G, Reid W, Burns G (1977): Fetal malnutrition: an appraisal of correlated factors. Am J Obstet Gynecol 128:22–31.

Darby WJ, McGanity WJ, Martin MP, Bridgforth E, Densen PM, Kaser MM, Ogle PL, Newbill JA, Stockell A, Ferguson ME, Touster I, McClellan GS, Williams C, Cannon RO (1953): The Vanderbilt cooperative study of maternal and infant nutrition. IV. Dietary. Laboratory and physical findings in 2,129 delivered pregnancies. J Nutr 51: 565–97.

Davies DP, Gray OP, Ellwood PC, Abernethy M (1976): Cigarette smoking in pregnancy: associations with maternal weight gain and fetal growth. Lancet 1:385–7.

Dobbing J, Sands J (1973): Quantitative growth and development of the human brain. Arch Dis Child 48:757–67.

Dobbing J, Smart JL (1973): Early undernutrition, brain development and behavior. In Barnett SA (ed): "Clinics in Developmental Medicine, No. 47: Ethology and Development." London: William Heinemann, pp 16–36.

Douglas JWB (1960): "Premature" children at primary schools. Br Med J 1:1008–13.

Drillien CM (1964): "The Growth and Development of the Prematurely Born Infant." Baltimore: Williams & Wilkins.

Drillien CM (1972): Aetiology and outcome in low-birthweight infants. Dev Med Child Neurol 14:563–74.

Feldman JF, Brody N (1978): Non-elicited newborn behavior in relation to state and prandial condition. Merrill-Palmer Q 24:79–84.

Food and Nutritional Board, National Academy of Sciences, National Research Council (1974): "Recommended Dietary Allowances." Washington, D.C.: 8th Revision.

Frankova S (1974): Interactions between early malnutrition and stimulation in animals. In Cravioto J, Hambraeus L, Vahlquist B (eds): "Symposia of the Swedish Nutrition Foundation. XII: Early Malnutrition and Mental Development." Uppsala: Almqvist & Wiksell, pp 202–10.

Frankova S (1978): Effect of malnutrition and early environment on behavioral development and long-term mental disturbances in rats. In Mittler P (ed): "Research to Practice in Mental Retardation: Volume III, Biomedical Aspects." Baltimore: University Park Press, pp 365–74.

Garber HL (1975): Intervention in infancy: a developmental approach. In Begab MJ, Richardson SA (eds): "The Mentally Retarded and Society: A Social Science Perspective." Baltimore: University Park Press, pp 287–304.

Gruenwald P (1966): Growth of the human fetus. I. Normal growth and its variation. Am J Obstet Gynecol 94:1112–9.

Habicht JP, Yarbrough C, Lechtig A, Klein RE (1974): Relation of maternal supplementary feeding during pregnancy to birthweight and other sociobiological factors. In Winick M (ed): "Proceedings of the Symposium on Nutrition and Fetal Development." New York: John Wiley & Sons, pp 127–46.

Hansen JDL, Freesemann C, Moodie AD, Evans DE (1971): What does nutritional growth retardation imply? Pediatrics 47 (Suppl): 299–313.

Herriot RM, Hsueh AM, Aitchison R (1978): "Influence of Maternal Diet on Offspring: Growth, Behavior, Feed Efficiency and Susceptibility (Human)." (A study in Suilin, Taiwan, initiated by Bacon F. Chow.) Final report on AID/CSD 2944 Contract with the John Hopkins University.

Hertzig MM, Birch HG, Richardson SA, Tizard J (1972): Intellectual levels of school children severely malnourished during the first two years of life. Pediatrics 49:814–24.

Hutt C (1968): Exploration of novelty in children with and without upper CNS lesions and some effects of auditory and visual incentives. Acta Psychol (Amst) 28:150–60.

Hytten FE, Leitch I (1971): "The Physiology of Human Pregnancy," 2nd Ed. Oxford: Blackwell Scientific Publications.

Kagan J (1971): "Change and Continuity in Infancy." New York: John Wiley & Sons.

Klein RE, Irwin M, Engle PL, Townsend J, Lechtig A, Martorell R, Delgado H (1977): Malnutrition, child health, and behavioural development. Data from an intervention study. In Mittler P (ed): "Research to Practice in Mental Retardation: Volume III, Biomedical Aspects." Baltimore: University Park Press, pp 299–310.

Koenigsberger MR (1966): Judgment of fetal age. I. Neurologic evaluation. Pediatr Clin North Am 13:823–33.

Langner TS, Herson JH, Greene EL, Jameson JD, Goff JA (1970): In Allen

VL (ed): "Psychological Factors in Poverty." Chicago: Markham, pp 185–209.

Lester BM (1975): Cardiac habituation of the orienting response to an auditory signal in infants of varying nutritional status. Dev Psychol 11:432–42.

Levitsky DA (1975): Maldevelopment and animal models of cognitive development. In Serban G (ed): "Advances in Behavioral Biology: Volume 14, Nutrition and Mental Functions." New York: Plenum Press, pp 75–89.

Lewis M (1971): Individual differences in the measurement of early cognitive growth. In Hellmuth J (ed): "Exceptional Infant, Studies in Abnormalities, Vol. 2." New York: Brunner-Mazel, pp 172–210.

McKay H, Sinisterra L, McKay A, Gomez H, Lloreda P (1978): Improving cognitive ability in chronically deprived children. Science 200: 270–8.

McKeown T (1970): Prenatal and early postnatal influences on measured intelligence. Br Med J 3:63–7.

McKeown T, Record RG (1953): The influence of placental size on foetal growth in man, with special reference to multiple pregnancy. J Endocrinol 9:418–26.

Mantel N, Haenszel W (1959): Statistical aspects of data from retrospective studies of disease. J Natl Cancer Inst 22:719–48.

Metcoff J (1978): Association of fetal growth with maternal nutrition. In Falkner F, Tanner JM (eds): "Human Growth. A Comprehensive Treatise." New York: Plenum Press, pp 415–60.

Milner RDG, Richards B (1974): An analysis of birth weight by gestation age of infants born in England and Wales, 1967–71. J Obstet Gynecol Br Commonweal 81:956–67.

Mora JO, Clement J, Christiansen N, Ortiz N, Vuori L, Wagner M, Herrera MG (1977): Nutritional supplementation, early home stimulation, and child development. Paper presented at International Conference on Behavioral Effects of Energy and Protein Deficits, Washington, D.C.

Mora JO, de Paredes B, Wagner M, de Navarro L, Suescon J, Christiansen N, Herrera MG (1979): Nutritional supplementation and the outcome of pregnancy. I. Birthweight. Am J Clin Nutr 32 (2): 455–62.

Neligan GA, Kevin I, Scott D McI, Garside RF (1976): "Born Too Soon or Born Too Small: A Follow-Up Study to Seven Years of Age." Philadelphia: J.B. Lippincott.

Nuchpakdee M (1978): Spared brain growth in human intrauterine growth retardation. Doctoral Dissertation, Faculty of Medicine, Columbia University.

Pasamanick B, Knobloch H (1966): Retrospective studies of the epidemiology of reproductive casualty: old and new. Merrill-Palmer Q 12:7–26.

Pederson FA, Wender PH (1968): Early social correlates of cognitive functioning in six year old boys. Child Dev 39:185–94.

Pereira MG (1977): Effects of nutritional supplementation on biochemical parameters of the placenta. Doctoral Dissertation, Faculty of Medicine, Columbia University.

Ravelli G–P, Stein ZA, Susser MW (1976): Obesity in young men after famine exposure in utero and early infancy. N Engl J Med 295: 349–53.

Record RG, McKeown T, Edwards JH (1969a): The relation of measured intelligence to birth weight and duration of gestation. Ann Hum Genet 33:71–9.

Record RG, McKeown T, Edwards JH (1969b): The relation of measured intelligence to birth order and maternal age. Ann Hum Genet 33:61–9.

Richardson SA (1976): The relation of severe malnutrition in infancy to the intelligence of school children with differing life histories. Pediatr Res 10:57–61.

Riopelle AJ, Favrett R (1977): Protein deprivation in primates. XIII. Growth of infants born of deprived mothers. Hum Biol 49:321–33.

Riopelle AJ, Hale PA (1975): Nutritional and environmental factors affecting gestation length in rhesus monkeys. Am J Clin Nutr 28: 1170–6.

Riopelle AJ, Hale PA, Watts ES (1976): Protein deprivation in primates. VII. Determinants of size and skeletal maturity at birth in rhesus monkeys. Hum Biol 48:203–22.

Riopelle AJ, Hill CW, Li S–C (1975): Protein deprivation in primates. V. Fetal mortality and neonatal status of infant monkeys born of deprived mothers. Am J Clin Nutr 28:989–93.

Riopelle AJ, Hill CW, Li S–C, Wolf RH, Seibold HR, Smith JL (1975): Protein deprivation in primates. IV. Pregnant rhesus monkey. Am J Clin Nutr 28:20–8.

Rush D (1972): Perinatal mortality, race, social status, and hospital of birth: the association with birthweight. In Janerich DT, Skalko RG, Porter IH (eds): "Symposium on Congenital Defects, New Directions in Research." New York: Academic Press, pp 161–9.

Rush D (1974): Examination of the relationship between birthweight, cigarette smoking during pregnancy, and maternal weight gain. J Obstet Gynecol Br Commonweal 81:746–52.

References

Rush D, Davis H, Susser M (1972): Antecedents of low birthweight in Harlem, New York City. Int J Epidemiol I:393–405.

Rush D, Higgins AC, Sadow MD, Margolis S (1976): Dietary services during pregnancy, and birthweight: a retrospective matched pair analysis (abstract). Pediatr Res 10:349.

Rush D, Stein Z, Christakis G, Susser M (1974): The Prenatal Project: the first 20 months of operation. In Winick M (ed): "Nutrition and Fetal Development." New York: John Wiley & Sons, pp 95–125.

Sindram IS (1945): De invloed van andervoeding op de groei van de vrücht. Ned T Verlosk 45:30–48.

Skodak M, Skeels HM (1945): A follow-up study of children in adoptive homes. J Genet Psychol 66:21–58.

Smith CA (1947): Effects of wartime starvation in Holland on pregnancy and its products. Am J Obstet Gynecol 54:599–608.

Stein Z, Kassab H (1970): Nutrition. In Wortis J (ed): "Mental Retardation, Vol II." New York: Grune & Stratton, pp 92–116.

Stein ZA, Susser MW (1975a): The Dutch famine, 1944/45 and the reproductive process. I. Effects on six indices at birth. Pediatr Res 9: 70–6.

Stein ZA, Susser MW (1975b): The Dutch famine, 1944/45, and the reproductive process. II. Interrelations of caloric rations and six indices at birth. Pediatr Res 9:76–83.

Stein Z, Susser M, Saenger G, Marolla F (1975): "Famine and Human Development: The Dutch Hunger Winter of 1944/45." New York: Oxford University Press.

Stein Z, Susser M, Rush D (1978): Prenatal nutrition and birthweight: experiments and quasi-experiments in the past decade. J Reprod Med 21:287–99.

Stroink J (1947): De duur der zwangerschap en het gewicht der neonati in de hongerperiode 1944-45. Ned T Verlosk 47:101–5.

Susser M (1973): "Causal Thinking in the Health Sciences: Concepts and Strategies in Epidemiology." New York: Oxford University Press.

Susser MW, Marolla FA, Fleiss J (1972): Birthweight, fetal age and perinatal mortality. Am J Epidemiol 96:197–204.

Thomson AM (1959): 3. Diet in relation to the course and outsome of pregnancy. Br J Nutr 13:509–25.

Turkewitz G, Moreau T, Birch HG (1968): Relation between birth condition and neuro-organization in the neonate. Pediatr Res 2:243–9.

U.S. Department of Health, Education and Welfare Publication (1972): Nos. (HSM) 72-8240-8134, "The Ten-State Nutrition Survey, 1968–70." Washington, D.C.: Government Printing Office.

Usher R, McLean F, Scott KE (1966): Judgment of fetal age. II. Clinical significance of gestational age and an objective method for its assessment. Pediatr Clin North Am 13:835–62.

Vuori L, Christiansen N, Clement J, Mora JO, Wagner M, Herrera MG (1979): Nutritional supplementation and the outcome of pregnancy. II. Visual habituation at 15 days. Am J Clin Nutr 32:463–9.

Wiener G (1970): The relationship of birthweight and length of gestation to intellectual development at ages 8 to 10 years. J Pediatr 76:693–99.

Wiener G, Rider RV, Oppel WC, Harper PH (1968): Correlates of low birth weight. Psychological status at eight to ten years of age. Pediatr Res 2:110–18.

Winick M, Noble A (1966): Cellular response in rats during malnutrition at various ages. J Nutr 89:300–6.

Wolff PH (1966): The causes, controls, and organization of behavior in the neonate. Psychol Issues 5:1–105.

Zamenhof S, van Marthens E, Margolis FL (1968): DNA (cell number) and protein in neonatal brain: alteration by maternal dietary protein restriction. Science 160:322–3.

Index

Affective states, and nutrition, 128–29
Age, maternal, 40, 41; see also Maternal characteristics
Aitchison, 52, 53, 84, 117, 118
Alkaline ribonuclease, 19
Apgar score, 18
Auditory stimulation, 92, 99

Barnes, 120
Bayley Scales, 90–91, 93, 96, 103, 118, 167–68
Belmont, 127
Bergner, 1, 2, 5, 101, 105, 115
Beverages, nutritional. See New York study, nutritional beverages
Birch, 1
Birthweight
  among blacks, 5
  in Bogotá study, 111–12
  conclusions about, in nutritional studies, 123–25
  and conditional effects, 72
  as dependent variable, 4
  design of study of, 1–25
  and diet intake, 153
  in Dutch famine study, 120–21
  in Guatemala study, 113–16
  low, 8, 59; see also Birthweight, past low
  and material calorie intake, 114, 115, 116
  and maternal nutrition, 1–3
  and maternal weight gain, 78, 109–10, 124
  in Montreal study, 108–10
  and multiple regression analysis, 72
  in New York study, 64–71, 77–85, 92, 107, 129–52
  and nutrition, 17, 124, 125
  and nutritional supplements, 85
  and past low birthweight, 47, 74, 82, 109
  and perinatal mortality, 1
  and protein, 4
  and smoking, 77, 83
  and social factors, 125
  and specific nutrients, 124, 125
  and supplements, 69, 123–32
  and vitamin C, 3
Blacks, 5, 107
Blackwell, 53, 117
Blanc, 18
Boelkins, 100, 102, 103, 130
Bogotá (Colombia) study, 102, 106, 110–12, 115, 116, 124, 130
  factorial design in, 110
  summary of, 172–77
Brody, 18

Calorie intake
  and birthweight, 114, 115, 116, 118, 124
  deficit in, 47, 53, 83, 108
  and fetal growth, 12n
  of groups in New York study, 36, 48
  and multiple regression analysis, 73
  and premature birth, 57
  /protein ratio, 102
  and weight gain, 45
Cape Town study. See South Africa study
Causal model, 88
Chavez, 127, 128

Child development, 1; *see also* Mental functions; Psychological measures; Somatic measures
Chinn, 117
Chow, 52, 84, 117
Complement group, New York study, 11, 12, 13, 24, 34, 36, 40, 47, 53
  and calorie intake, 48
  favorable effects in, 83
  and neonatal death, 60–61
  outcomes, 52n, 78–79
  protein amount in, 101
  weight gain in, 49
  see also New York study; Treatment, New York study
Control group, New York study, 11, 13, 24, 25, 34, 36, 40, 47, 48
  neonatal death in, 59–61
  outcomes, 78
  weight gain in, 49
  see also New York study; Treatment, New York study
Cord blood, 17, 18
Corman, 90
Cravioto, 127, 128
Crosby, 124

Darby, 3
Davis, 2, 107
DeLicardie, 127, 128
Diet, 24-hour recall. *See* New York study, diet recall, 24-hour
Dietary intake
  and birthweight, 83, 108, 153
  in Bogotá study, 112
  in Dutch famine study, 120
  and extreme prematurity, 57
  and fetal growth, 79
  in Guatemala study, 113
  and maternal weight gain, 54, 142
  in New York study, 30–41, 51
  in Taiwan study, 117
DNA, 19

Dobbing, 92, 122
Down syndrome, 20
Douglas, 1, 87
Drillien, 1, 87
Dutch famine study, 1, 2, 12n, 83, 87, 88, 106, 120–23, 125, 132
  psychological effects of starvation, 125
  summary of, 172–77

Education, maternal, 40, 81, 127
Edwards, 87
Environment, postnatal, 126–27
Escalona, 90
Evans, 18
Experiment
  natural, 105
  quasi, 105, 108, 114, 126
  see also specific studies

Factorial design, 110
Famine
  observational studies of, 3
  see also Dutch famine study
Favrett, 52, 84, 124
Fetal dimensions, in Dutch famine study, 121
Fetal growth
  and calorie intake, 12n
  in Dutch famine study, 121, 122
  and malnutrition, 126
  and maternal nutrition, 101
  and maternal weight gain, 77
  retardation of, and supplement, 69, 124
Fetal mortality
  definition of, 59
  and protein deprivation, 84
  and social attributes of mothers, 61, 63
  and treatment in New York study, 61, 62
Fetal weight gain
  and maternal smoking, 147–48

Fleiss, 1
Frankova, 92, 127, 129

Garber, 126
Gestation, duration of, 49, 52n
  associations of, 57
  and birthweight, 109
  in Dutch famine study, 121
  life table analysis, 55–56
  and maternal characteristics, 57–58, 61
  and multiple regression analysis, 72, 73
  and perinatal mortality, 1
  and treatment in New York study, 92
Growth, fetal. *See* Fetal growth
Gruenwald, 2
Guatemala study, 12n, 84, 99, 106, 112–17, 124–26, 129, 132
  psychological effects in, 126, 129
  regression analysis, 114
  self-selection in, 115
  summary of, 172–77
Gussow, 1

Habicht, 12n, 84, 106, 112
Haenszel, 55
Hale, 52, 84, 124
Hansen, 127, 129
Hegsted, 100, 102, 103, 130
Height, maternal, 2
Herriot, 52, 53, 84, 117, 118
Hertzig, 127, 128
Higgins, 108
High protein intake
  adverse effects of, 80–85, 97
  anorectic effect of, 82
  overload, 82
  in Rhesus monkeys, 84
  see also New York study, protein supplement in; Protein
Hill, 124
Hsueh, 52, 53, 84, 117, 118

Hutt, 100

Immunoglobulins, 18, 19
Infant, as stimulus to parent, 128–29
Intervention, nutritional. *See* Nutrition, intervention
Iron, 12

Jamaica, 127, 128

Kagan, 100
Klein, 129
Knobloch, 1
Koenigsberger, 19
Kwashiorkor, 128

Lester, 92,
Levitsky, 92
Lewis, 92, 99, 100, 103
Li, 124
Life table analysis of
  gestational duration, 55–56
  neonatal death rate, 59, 144
  prematurity, 143
Low birthweight. *See* Birthweight, low; Birthweight, past low

McKay, 126
McKeown, 1, 2, 87, 126
McLean, 19
Malnutrition, 125–28; *see also* Dutch famine study; Nutrition
Mantel, 55
Margolis, 12
Marolla, 1, 127
Martinez, 127
Maternal characteristics
  age, 40, 41
  and duration of gestation, 57–58, 61
  education, 40, 81, 127
  and fetal death, 61
  in Guatemala study, 115
  height, 2

and perinatal mortality, 63
and weight gain during pregnancy, 2
Maternal weight, preconception, 2
Maternal weight gain, 2
average, in New York study, 41, 44, 45, 47, 54
and birthweight, 78, 109–10, 124
in complement group, New York study, 78–79
correlations, 49
and dietary intake, 45–47
in Dutch famine study, 120–21
early, in New York study, 41, 44, 45, 47, 54, 81, 82, 138–39
of early entrants, in New York study, 50
and fetal dimensions, 79
and fetal growth, 77
indices, in New York study, 41–44, 54
interpretation of, in New York study, 50
low, 8
and low birthweight, 109–10
multiple regression analysis, 45–46
New York study data on, 135–42
and nutritional intervention, 49–52
and supplement group, in New York study, 44, 81–83, 111
total, in New York study, 41, 44, 45, 54
in treatment group, in New York study, 44, 92–93
Mature births
and birthweight, 67–69
mean birthweight in, 78
and protein-related measures, 102–3
and treatment, in New York study, 67–69
see also Premature births

Mental functions
outcome, in New York study, 87–104
and postnatal environment, 126–27
and social factors, 128–29
and somatic measures, 130
see also Psychological measures
Metabolism, 51
Metcoff, 124
Mexico study, 127–28, 177
Milner, 69n
Monkeys
visual habituation in, 100, 102, 103
see also Primates; Rhesus monkeys
Montreal Diet Dispensary, 108
Montreal study, 106, 108–10, 122, 123
summary of, 172–77
Mora, 106, 110, 112, 130
Mortality, fetal. See Fetal mortality,
Multiple regression analysis, New York Study
Bayley Scores, 96, 167–68
birthweight, 72, 149–53
calorie intake, 73
dietary intake, 142
gestational duration, 73
newborn dimensions, 73
play, 171
smoking, 73
visual dishabituation, 97, 170
visual habituation, 96–97, 169
weight gain, 140–41

Naeye, 18
Natural experiment, 105
Neligan, 1
Neonatal deaths, New York study
in complement group, 60
in control group, 59, 60
life table analysis, 59
and maternal attributes, 63
in supplement group, 59, 60, 81, 132

and treatment, 62, 65, 144–45
Newborn dimensions, New York
—— study, 61
  data, 147–48
  and dietary indices, 71–72
  and past low birthweight, 74
  and smoking, 73–74, 147–48
  and treatment, 71–72
New York study, 105–8, 110, 122–26
  anamnestic indices, 28–30, 32, 34
  attrition rate, 9, 19–20
  between-group differences, 77–78
  birthweight data, 149–53
  can count, 28, 30, 34
  causal model, 88
  complement group. See Complement group, New York study; Treatment, New York study
  conditional effects, 72
  consistency, 30
  control group. See Control group, New York study
  control of confounding, 96
  control variables, 72
  cord blood, 17, 18
  delivery data, 134
  design, 4–25
  diet, substitution of regular, 34–41
  diet gradients, 48, 50
  diet history, 28–29
  diet, 24-hour recall, 16, 27, 28
  dietary intake, 30–41, 49, 51
  double-blind study, 12
  enrollment, 9, 13, 16, 19–20
  entry cohort, 66, 67, 69
  fetal deaths, 59, 61–63
  fetal growth, 61, 69, 77, 101, 124, 147–48
  flow chart, 13
  gestational age, 4
  and gestational duration, 49, 52n 55–56, 61, 72–73, 92, 109

intervention, nutritional, 2, 4–13, 27–54, 147–48
life table analysis, 55–56, 59, 143–144
maternal smoking. See Smoking, maternal
maternal weight gain. See Maternal weight gain
mature births, 67–69, 78, 102–3
monitoring of intervention, 27–54
multiple regression analysis. See Multiple regression analysis, New York study
neonatal deaths. See Neonatal deaths, New York study
newborn dimensions. See Newborn dimensions, New York study
newborn maturity evaluation, 19
nutritional beverages, 9–13, 30–41
observed data, 30, 32
outcome, one year, 87–104
outcome, one year/adverse at birth, 102–3
pathological exam, 17, 18
perinatal mortality, 20, 25, 59–62, 85, 111, 116, 132
pilot experimental period, 13
placental studies, 17–19, 52n, 124, 178, 180
pregnancy data, 133
premature births data, 142
protein supplement in, 4, 8, 11–13, 16, 19, 36, 45, 47, 53, 101–2
psychological measures in, 89–91, 93–104, 108, 112, 116–118, 125–32, 154–157, 161–71
random assignment, 4, 8, 16
rationale for choice of measures, 91–92
recruitment, 9, 13, 16, 19–20

reliability, 30
replacements, 9
riboflavin in, 9, 12, 16, 29, 32, 34, 40, 45, 49, 51–52
sample size, 5
selection criteria, 5–9
serum vitamin levels, 16–18
social history, 17–18
somatic measures in. *See* Somatic measures
statistical power, 98–99
stratification, 4, 8, 16
summary of, 172–77
supplement group. *See* Supplement group, New York study; Treatment, New York study
target population, 5–9, 47, 53
testing procedures in, 89–91; *see also* New York study, psychological measures; Somatic measures
treatment. *See* Treatment, New York study
weight gain data, 135–42; *see also* Maternal weight gain
within-group differences, 78–80
Noble, 12, 120
Nutrition
and affective states, 128–29
and birthweight, 3
conclusions about prenatal, 123–32
controlled trials in study of, 105
deprivation, effects of, 125–26
and fetal growth, 1, 101
and infant affective states, 129
intervention, in Bogotá study, 110–12
intervention, in Montreal study, 108–10
intervention, in New York study, 2, 9–13, 27–41, 147–48
and maternal affective states, 128
and social factors, 128–29, 131
and somatic effects, 129

studies of, 3–4; 105–23; *see also* Bogotá study; Dutch famine study; Guatemala study; Mexico study; Montreal study; New York study; South Africa study; Taiwan study
see also Supplementation

Obesity, 122, 125
Object permanence, 91, 93, 103

Parents, infant as stimulus to, 128–29
Pasamanick, 1
Pederson, 100
Perinatal mortality
and birthweight, 116
in Guatemala study, 116
and maternal nutritional deprivation, 122
and maternal nutritional supplementation, 85
in New York study, 20, 25, 59–62, 85, 111, 116, 132
and race, 1, 5
and social status, 1
Placenta
biochemical analysis of, 17–19, 52n, 124, 178
growth, and maternal weight gain, 124
histomorphometry, 18–19, 178
histopathology of, 180
weight, in Dutch famine study, 121
Play, 90–91, 93, 95, 97–98, 100, 103, 171
Postnatal environment, 126–27
Pregnancy
appetite during, 115
New York study data on, 133
see also Gestation
Premature births
birthweight of, in Bogotá study, 112
birthweight of, in New York

study, 78
and dietary intake, 57
and growth-related measures, 102
and high protein supplement. *See* premature births, and supplement
and perinatal mortality, 1
and size at one year, 93
and supplement, 54, 56–60, 66, 69, 80–81, 102–3, 125
and treatment, in New York study, 97, 104, 143
see also Mature births
Primates, 130; *see also* Monkeys; Rhesus monkeys
Protein
adequacy of, 108
adverse effects of prenatal, 123–24
and birthweight, 4, 118
/calorie ratio, 102
deprivation, 11–12, 16, 47, 53
in Guatemala study, 113–14
intake, in New York study, 4, 8, 36
level at birth, 19
and maternal weight gain, 45
place of, in prenatal diet, 125
and premature births, 57, 66, 125
related measures, 95, 98–99, 102–4, 108, 126, 130–32
and psychological development, 108, 131–32
see also High protein intake; New York study, protein supplement in
Psychological measures
in Bogotá study, 112
conclusions about, in nutritional studies, 125–32
correlation with somatic measures, 155–57

description of, 90–91
and growth, 95, 97–99, 102–4, 130–31
in Guatemala study, 116, 126, 129
at one year, in New York study, 154, 161–71
outcome, in New York study, 93–104, 154, 161–71
protein-related, 95, 98–99, 102–4, 108, 126, 130–32
and starvation, 22–23, 125
and supplement, in New York study, 112, 116–18
testing of, 89
and treatment, in New York study, 93–104
in Taiwan study, 126
see also Mental functions
Psychosocial stimulation, 110

Quasi experiment, 105, 108, 114, 126
Quetelet's index, 20

Race, 1; *see also* Blacks
Ravelli, 122
Raven's Progressive Matrices, 122
RDA (Recommended Dietary Allowance), 47
Record, 2, 52, 87, 126
Regression analysis
in Guatemala study, 114
in New York study. *See* Multiple regression analysis, New York study
Reliability, index, 30n
Rhesus monkeys, 84, 124; *see also* Monkeys
Riboflavin. *See* New York study, riboflavin
Richards, 69n
Richardson, 127, 128
Riopelle, 52, 84, 124
RNA, 19
Rush, 1, 2, 5, 107, 108

Sands, 122
Scott, 19
Self-selection, in nutritional studies, 115, 118
Sever, John, 18
Sex differences
　in birthweight, 112, 115
　and intrauterine nutrition, 125
Sindram, 120
Sinisterra, 126
Skeels, 126
Skodak, 126
Smart, 92
Smith, 101, 120
Smoking, maternal, 2, 8–9, 40, 85, 112
　and birthweight, 77, 83, 107
　multiple regression analysis, 73
　and newborn dimensions, 73–74, 147–48
　and supplement, in New York Study, 73, 107, 123, 124
Social factors and
　birthweight, 125
　cognitive ability, 126–27
　fetal death, 61
　malnutrition, 128
　mental capability, 128
　nutrition, 131
　prenatal mortality, 1
　protein intake, 12
Somatic measures
　correlation with psychological measures, 130, 155–57
　description of, 90
　maternal predictors of, 95
　and nutrition, 129
　at one year old, 158–60
　outcome, in New York study, 93
　and supplement, in New York study, 113
　testing of, 89

and treatment, in New York study, 92–93, 95, 103–4
South Africa study, 127, 129
Stanford-Binet tests, 92, 99
Starvation. *See* Dutch famine study
Stein, 1, 2, 12n, 83, 87, 101, 106, 115, 120, 122, 127
Stroink, 120
Supplementation, prenatal, in Bogotá study, 110–12
Supplementation, prenatal, in Guatemala study, 112–17
Supplementation, prenatal, in New York study, 27–28, 51–52
　beverage form of, 9–13, 16, 28, 34
　and birthweight, 1–2
　as independent variable, 4
　monitoring of, 10, 27–54
　nutrient composition, 10
　one year outcome, 87–104
　and perinatal mortality, 132
　and smoking, 123–24
Supplementation, prenatal, in Taiwan study, 117–19
Supplement group, New York study
　adverse effects of, 80–85, 97, 102–3
　beneficial effect, 104
　and birthweight, 59, 69, 107
　calorie intake by, 48
　dissociation of, on maternal weight gain, 77
　entry cohorts, 40
　and growth retardation, 69
　and maternal weight gain, 44–47, 49, 54
　and mental function, 99
　monitoring of intake by, 36, 48
　and neonatal deaths, 59–61, 132

outcome, 103–4
and premature births, 56–59
protein amount in, 4, 11, 12, 13, 101–2
and psychological measures, 94–95, 131–32
and smoking, 73, 123, 124
and superior mental function, 99
and visual habituation/dishabituation, 130
see also New York study; Supplementation, prenatal, in New York study; Treatment, New York study
Susser, 1, 2, 5, 96, 101, 105, 107, 115, 120, 122, 127

Taiwan study, 117–19, 126
psychological effects of, 126
self-selection in, 118
summary of, 172–77
Ten State Nutritional Survey, 28
Thomson, 3, 83, 115
Treatment, New York study
adherence to, 28–30, 47
and Bayley Scores, 167–68
and birthweight, 64–71, 149–52
conditional nature of effects, 52, 92
entry, early, 81, 82
entry cohort, 44
entry, time of, 92
effects, 52, 83, 92
favorable effect of, 83
groups, 5, 20–24; *see also* Complement group, New York study; Control group, New York study; Supplement group, New York study
and maternal weight gain, 135–41
and maturity, 44, 67–69, 70

and neonatal deaths, 65, 144–45
and newborn dimensions, 71, 147–48
and placenta, 178
and play, 171
and prematurity, 44, 56, 143
and visual habituation/dishabituation, 169–70

Urinary riboflavin assay. *See* New York study, riboflavin
Usher, 19
Uzgiris-Hunt measure, 90

Validity, index, 30n
Van Marthens, 12
Visual dishabituation, in New York study, 91, 93–95, 97–98, 103–4, 130
Visual habituation
in Bogotá study, 112
and high protein supplement, 103
in New York study, 90–100, 103–4, 130, 169
and nutritional deprivation, 126
and primates, 130
of young infants, 103
Vitamin C, 3
Voori, 99

Watts, 52, 84, 124
Wechsler Intelligence Scale, 100
Weight gain, fetal. *See* Fetal weight gain
Weight, maternal. *See* Maternal weight; Maternal weight gain
Wender, 100
Wiener, 1, 87
Winick, 12, 18, 120

Zamenhof, 12
Zinc, 11

BOOKS PUBLISHED BY ALAN R. LISS, INC. FOR THE NATIONAL FOUNDATION

BIRTH DEFECTS: ORIGINAL ARTICLE SERIES

1975 — Volume XI

No. 7   **Morphogenesis and Malformation of Face and Brain,** Daniel Bergsma and Jan Langman, *Editors*

1976 — Volume XII

No. 1   **Cancer and Genetics,** Daniel Bergsma, R. Neil Schimke, Robert L. Summitt, and David J. Harris, *Editors*

No. 3   **The Eye and Inborn Errors of Metabolism,** Daniel Bergsma, Anthony J. Bron and Edward Cotlier, *Editors*

No. 4   **Developmental Disabilities: Psychologic and Social Implications,** Daniel Bergsma and Ann E. Pulver, *Editors*

No. 5   **Cytogenetics, Environment and Malformation Syndromes,** Daniel Bergsma and R. Neil Schimke, *Editors*

No. 6   **Growth Problems and Clinical Advances,** Daniel Bergsma and R. Neil Schimke, *Editors*

No. 8   **Iron Metabolism and Thalassemia,** Daniel Bergsma, Anthony Cerami, Charles M. Peterson, and Joseph H. Graziano, *Editors*

1977 — Volume XIII

No. 1   **Morphogenesis and Malformation of the Limb,** Daniel Bergsma and Widukind Lenz, *Editors*

No. 2   **Morphogenesis and Malformation of the Genital System,** Richard J. Blandau and Daniel Bergsma, *Editors*

No. 3   **Annual Review of Birth Defects, 1976,** Daniel Bergsma and R. Brian Lowry, *Editors*
Proceedings of the 1976 Vancouver Birth Defects Conference. Published in 4 volumes:
   3A   **Numerical Taxonomy of Birth Defects** *and* **Polygenic Disorders**
   3B   **New Syndromes**
   3C   **Natural History of Specific Birth Defects**
   3D   **Embryology and Pathogenesis** *and* **Prenatal Diagnosis**

No. 5   **Urinary System Malformations in Children,** Daniel Bergsma and John W. Duckett, *Editors*

No. 6   **Trends and Teaching in Clinical Genetics,** Daniel Bergsma, Frederick Hecht, Gerald H. Prescott, and Joan H. Marks, *Editors*

1978 — Volume XIV

No. 1   **Genetic Effects on Aging,** Daniel Bergsma and David E. Harrison, *Editors*

No. 2   **The Molecular Basis of Cell-Cell Interaction,** Richard A. Lerner and Daniel Bergsma, *Editors*

No. 3 **The Genetics of Hand Malformations,** *by* Samia A. Temtamy and Victor A. McKusick
No. 5 **Neurochemical and Immunologic Components in Schizophrenia,** Daniel Bergsma and Allan L. Goldstein, *Editors*
No. 6 **Annual Review of Birth Defects, 1977,** Robert L. Summitt and Daniel Bergsma, *Editors*
Proceedings of the 1977 Memphis Birth Defects Conference. Published in 3 volumes:
  6A Cell Surface Factors, Immune Deficiencies, Twin Studies
  6B Recent Advances *and* New Syndromes
  6C Sex Differentiation *and* Chromosomal Abnormalities
No. 7 **Morphogenesis and Malformation of the Cardiovascular System,** Glenn C. Rosenquist and Daniel Bergsma, *Editors*

1979 — Volume XV

No. 1 **Sex Chromosome Aneuploidy: Prospective Studies on Children,** Arthur Robinson, Herbert A. Lubs, and Daniel Bergsma, *Editors*
No. 2 **Genetic Counseling: Facts, Values, and Norms,** Alexander M. Capron, Marc Lappé, Robert F. Murray, Jr., Tabitha M. Powledge, Sumner B. Twiss, and Daniel Bergsma, *Editors*
No. 3 **Recent Advances in the Developmental Biology of Central Nervous System Malformation,** Ntinos C. Myrianthopoulos and Daniel Bergsma, *Editors*
No. 4 **Continuous Transcutaneous Blood Gas Monitoring,** A. Huch, R. Huch, and J. Lucey, *Editors*
No. 5 **Annual Review of Birth Defects, 1978,** Proceedings of the 1978 San Francisco Birth Defects Conference. Published in 3 volumes:
  5A **Diagnostic Approaches to the Malformed Fetus, Abortus, Stillborn, and Deceased Newborn,** Mitchell S. Golbus and Bryan D. Hall, *Editors*
  5B **Penetrance and Variability in Malformation Syndromes,** James J. O'Donnell and Bryan D. Hall, *Editors*
  5C **Risks, Communication, and Decision Making in Genetic Counseling,** Charles J. Epstein, Cynthia J.R. Curry, Seymour Packman, Sanford Sherman, and Bryan D. Hall, *Editors*
No. 6 **Dermatoglyphics — Fifty Years Later,** Wladimir Wertelecki and Chris C. Plato, *Editors*
No. 7 **Newborn Behavioral Organization: Nursing Research and Implications,** Gene Cranston Anderson and Beverly Raff, *Editors*
No. 8 **Developmental Aspects of Craniofacial Dysmorphology,** Michael Melnick and Ronald Jorgenson, *Editors*
No. 9 **External Ear Malformations: Epidemiology, Genetics, and Natural History,** by Michael Melnick and Ntinos C. Myrianthopoulos